Shades of Life

One Destination
Multiple Approaches
What's Yours?

Dr. T. S. Parmar

Copyright © 2024 by Dr. T. S. Parmar

All rights reserved.

This book or any portion thereof may not be reproduced or used in any manner whatsoever without the express written permission of the respective writer of the respective content except for the use of brief quotations in a book review.

The writer of the respective work holds sole responsibility for the originality of the content and The Write Order is not responsible in any way whatsoever.

Printed in India

ISBN: 978-93-6045-357-2

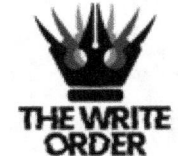

First Printing, 2024

The Write Order

A division of Pratilipi

Koramangala, Bangalore

Karnataka-560029

THE WRITE ORDER PUBLICATIONS.

www.thewriteorder.com

Content Curator: Anagha Somanakoppa

Typeset by Parinkumar Nirmal

Book Cover designed by Sankhasubhro Nath

Publishing Consultant: Anagha Somanakoppa

Acknowledgment & Dedication

My Book is Dedicated to

- ★ Widespread, adoption and perseverance of the 'values of human life' in today's disruptive world.

My Gratitude to

- ★ Almighty God.
- ★ My Parents, Parents-in-law, Elders, Gurus/Teachers.

My Acknowledgment and thanks to

- ★ The Write Order (Pratilipi & Westland Books) Team.
- ★ All who supported in the completion & launch of this book.
- ★ All Friends & Well wishers.

My Love and prayers for

- ★ My Family - Amanjyot (Wife), Angad (Son), Simran (Daughter), and Zen (Son-in-law).
- ★ My Siblings & their family.
- ★ Brother-in-law & his family.

First Impressions

𝒯he book front cover image was shared with the individuals listed below, and they were invited to share their initial impressions. I extend my sincere gratitude to each of these valued respondents for their delightful and encouraging feedback. I am confident that you, too, will find pleasure in reading through each of these responses, which are presented in alphabetical order based on the respondent's first name.

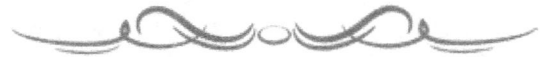

☆ Whatever my destination, personal or professional, it is having the right values and behaviors that have enabled me to reach where I am today. The ability to have good values and demonstrate them in my daily interactions has maximized value creation in every sphere of my life.

- **Anil Matai**
Director General, Organization of Pharmaceutical Producers of India (OPPI)
Former MD, Zydus Healthcare Ltd., and CEO, Novartis India Ltd.

✯ The cover of Shades of Life, at first glance, appears esoteric. But once you juxtapose the title of the book with the visual, it opens up delightful intrigue and whets the curiosity about what the contents could be. Given Dr. Parmar's deep study of human responses to multifarious life situations, this should make for a fascinating read.

- Ayaz Memon
Indian sports writer, journalist, columnist, author, and former lawyer.

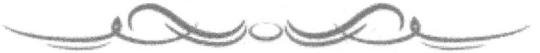

✯ Dr. Parmar takes a poignant topic and weaves magic with his words. Simple yet profound. A must read for anyone who is beginning his journey or standing at the crossroads of life. Unmissable!

- Cyrus F. Dastur
Founder, SHAMIANA
Asia's largest Short Film Platform

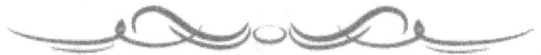

✯ I have no sympathy for the virtuous loser. Seeing his trampled example, people get dissuaded from the good path. Tony is a good man who has won—in the real world.Which is why I unhesitatingly recommend the maxims he presents in this insightful book. Must read for good guys who wish to triumph!

- Pavan Choudary
Bestselling Author, Business Leader, and Coach

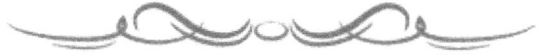

★ Tony Parmar brings rich life experiences to fruition with a book that will serve as a guide and inspiration to many. In an age where people's lives are being disrupted by tectonic changes, how does one hold onto core values? Shades of Life offers you a compass to a value-based journey.

- Rajdeep Sardesai
Senior Journalist and Author

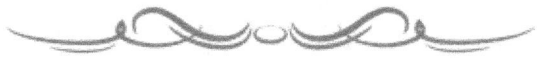

★ Life is unpredictable but beautiful. There are different shades of life, it is up to us to see what we want to see life as. The title of the book by Dr. Parmar forces every responsible person to think about the purpose and shades of life from their perspectives.

- Dr. Sanjeev Bansal
Dean FMS & Director ABS
Amity University Uttar Pradesh, Noida

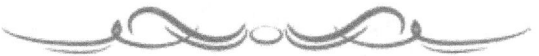

★ Excellent subject for all generations and is timeless. This will provide conceptual clarity with contextual familiarity in today's world.

- Sudarshan Jain
Secretary General,
India Pharmaceutical Alliance (IPA),
Former MD, Abbott Healthcare Ltd, India

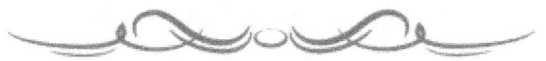

Table of Contents

	Prologue	1
1.	New Beginnings and Precious Arrivals	5
2.	Shades of Character	23
3.	Paths Diverge	39
4.	Paths of Transformation	57
5.	Whispers of the Heart	67
6.	Entangled Hearts	73
7.	Navigating Emotions	81
8.	Crossroads of Destiny	89
9.	Professionally Unraveled	97
10.	Celebration of Bonds	103
11.	Milestones and Unveiled Journeys	111
12.	Harmony in Choices	117
13.	A Journey into Life Coaching	123
14.	Rooted in Love	127
15.	Beyond Biology	135
	Concluding Note	139
	Epilogue	143
	About the Author	145

Prologue

Step into the enchanting world of these narratives, where life's intricate tapestry unfolds before you, each thread tinted with the vibrant hues of individual experiences. In this journey, you're not just a reader; you're a navigator, exploring the labyrinth of personal and professional dimensions and encountering a spectrum of personalities that reflect the diverse mosaic of human existence.

These tales are more than words on paper; they are open invitations to delve into the very essence of the human soul, to resonate with the ebbs and flows of joy, to face the challenges head-on, and to savor the triumphant moments that define our distinctive paths. Within the pages, you'll meet characters entangled in the intricate dance of love, striving for ambitious goals, navigating the complexities of family dynamics, and embarking on quests for purpose and fulfillment. Each character mirrors a facet of life, offering you a chance not just to read but to connect, empathize, and quite possibly see a reflection of yourself.

Mumbai, in the 20th Century, was a vibrant and bustling city, full of energy and rapid development. Known as Bombay at the time, it was the financial and commercial hub of India. The city was undergoing significant transformations, both economically and culturally. It was a time of industrial growth and urbanization, with many multinational corporations establishing their presence in Mumbai. The city's textile mills were thriving, contributing

Shades of Life

to its position as the textile capital of India.

Three lives, destined to intertwine, began their journey amidst the backdrop of 20th Century. Born into distinct families, each child brought with them a promise of untapped potential, their futures awaiting them like blank canvases eager to be painted upon.

In the quiet abode of a wise professor, a tiny bundle of joy emerged into the world. A child of curiosity and endless wonder, their future sparkled with the shimmering glow of knowledge and enlightenment. Oh, the dreams that swirled within the professor's heart, envisioning a legacy of wisdom passed down from generation to generation. As the professor held the baby in his arms, a deep sense of responsibility and awe engulfed him, knowing that this child possessed the power to change the world through the pursuit of knowledge.

Across town, in the bustling home of a prosperous businessman, another newborn made it's grand entrance. Surrounded by opulence and ambition, this little one was destined to inherit a legacy of entrepreneurship and financial prowess. In the eyes of the businessman, a flicker of hope ignited, envisioning a future where their offspring would carry the torch of success and elevate the family's name to new heights. The weight of expectation mingled with an intoxicating sense of possibility as the businessman cradled the baby, believing that they would shape the destiny of their lineage through the art of commerce.

And in the polished corridors of corporate professionals, a third family celebrated the arrival of their own precious gift. Born into a world of strategy and ambition, this child was destined to traverse the labyrinthine path of corporate success. The parents, acutely aware of the sacrifices and dedication demanded by their chosen profession, saw in their newborn the embodiment of their own aspirations and ambitions. Holding their baby close, they felt a blend of pride and anticipation, knowing their child would one day soar among the ranks of industry giants.

Oh, how fate weaves its tapestry, connecting the lives of these three babies, whose stories unfold in the chapters yet to be written. Their futures lay before them, a canvas begging for the brushstrokes of passion, dedication, and resilience. From the professor's abode, the businessman's mansion, and the corridors of corporate power, the world eagerly awaits the unfolding of these lives, bound by the threads of 20th Century, forever entwined in a tale of possibilities.

So, join us on this literary odyssey, traverse the varied landscapes of these lives, and let yourself be immersed in the collective symphony of emotions that binds us all. These stories are an exploration, an adventure, and an opportunity to unravel the universal threads that weave us together in the grand human experience.

Shades of Life

Chapter 1
New Beginnings and Precious Arrivals

"In the journey of life, each new beginning is a thread of hope, and every precious arrival is a masterpiece woven with the threads of joy, love, and boundless possibilities."

Family 1

In the bustling city of Bombay, a humble abode was home to a dedicated government teacher, Mr. Sharma. Within the confines of his small apartment, he nurtured a passion for education that burned brighter than any adversity he faced. The trials beset him on his journey as he tirelessly strived to make ends meet. Despite the harsh realities of financial constraint, Mr. Sharma's spirit remained unyielding, steadfast in his commitment to his principles. Day after day, he stepped into the classroom, his heart brimming with unwavering dedication. The weight of his own struggles never hindered his ability to impart knowledge to his eager students. He poured his soul into each lesson, igniting sparks of curiosity and illuminating young minds.

As the world outside spun in its relentless whirlwind, Mr. Sharma stood tall, a beacon of resilience amidst the storm. He understood the profound impact that education held, not just for the fortunate few but for every soul yearning to rise above their circumstances. Through his unwavering belief in the transformative power of learning, he carried a torch of hope that illuminated the path for his students, guiding them toward a brighter future. Though the financial burdens pressed heavily upon his shoulders, Mr. Sharma refused to let them extinguish his flame. His dedication, born from a love for his students and an unyielding passion for education, propelled him forward, undeterred by the shadows that loomed over his own life. In his eyes, every lesson delivered, every mind inspired, held the potential to shape a better tomorrow.

In the sanctuary of their shared home, Mr. Sharma and his beloved bride began a new chapter of their lives as husband and wife. Bound together by love and understanding, their hearts danced in harmony, creating a tapestry of affection that wove them ever closer. In the tender embrace of his wife, Mr. Sharma found solace and strength. Her unwavering support and understanding were like a soothing balm for his weary soul. Through every challenge they faced, their love endured, a beacon of warmth and companionship that illuminated even the darkest of days.

Financial hurdles often cast their shadows upon their path, especially when Mr. Sharma extended his helping hand to his students. But his wife, with a heart overflowing with love and respect, embraced his altruistic nature. She recognized the depths of his passion for teaching and the indomitable spirit that drove him to go that extra mile. Together, they weathered the storms of financial strain, knowing that the rewards of impacting young lives far outweighed any temporary setbacks. Amidst the ebb and flow of life's challenges, Mr. Sharma and his wife dreamt of expanding their loving union. They longed to bring a new life into their world, to nurture and cherish a child who would carry their love and values into the future. With each passing day, their anticipation grew as they prepared their home, their hearts brimming with hope and excitement.

In the tender moments of anticipation, Mrs. Sharma revealed the most precious news to her beloved husband, Mr. Sharma. A radiant smile illuminated her face as she whispered the words that would forever transform their lives—she was carrying their future within her womb. Joy, like a gentle symphony, echoed through their hearts, filling their souls with an overwhelming sense of happiness and love. From that moment forward, Mr. Sharma embraced his role with unwavering dedication and tenderness. Every waking hour became an opportunity for him to shower his beloved wife with care and affection. He witnessed the miracle of life unfolding within her, an awe-inspiring journey that left him in awe of the strength and beauty she possessed.

For nine transformative months, Mr. Sharma stood as a pillar of support, ensuring that every need of his wife was met. He eagerly attended every medical appointment, his heart brimming with a mixture of excitement and trepidation. He lovingly prepared nourishing meals, gently massaged her tired feet, and whispered words of love and encouragement to the precious life growing within. The bond deepened between them during those months! As he felt their child's first fluttering kicks against his hand, a profound sense of awe washed over Mr. Sharma. He understood the immense responsibility that awaited him, the privilege of guiding and protecting this tiny, vulnerable soul entrusted to their care.

In the quiet of their home, Mr. Sharma would sit beside his wife, his hand resting gently upon her growing belly. He would share stories and dreams, both for their child and for the life they would build together as a family. Each passing day brought them closer to the moment when their love would manifest itself in the form of their precious bundle of joy. As the countdown drew near, Mr. Sharma's heart overflowed with a kaleidoscope of emotions—anticipation, nervousness, and overwhelming love that transcended words. He knew that the world they had known was about to change forever, that their lives would be touched by a profound sense of wonder and responsibility.

Shades of Life

Outside the hospital door, a world of anticipation unfolded for Mr. Sharma, his heart both hopeful and anxious. His hard-earned savings had finally granted him the blessing he had longed for—a child of his own. With bated breath, he awaited the news, yearning to hear that both mother and baby were safe, their lives intertwined in love and joy. In Mr. Sharma's soul, there existed no distinction between the genders. For he had witnessed firsthand the injustices that befell his own sister, and in her struggles, he had found the seeds of compassion and empathy. To him, a boy and a girl were equal, deserving of equal opportunities and a world unburdened by prejudice.

As he stood outside the hospital, his mind wandered to the dreams he harbored for his unborn child. It was not riches or material possessions that he desired to bestow but a treasure far more profound—the gift of ideology and principled living. He yearned to raise his children not as mere products of society but as compassionate, resilient souls who would embrace the power of kindness and stand up against injustice. For Mr. Sharma, fatherhood was not a chance to enforce expectations upon his child but an opportunity to nurture and guide. He envisioned a world where his children would grow to be strong individuals, unyielding in their pursuit of truth and justice. He wanted them to understand that the power to effect change lay not in grand gestures but in the everyday choices they made, the empathy they showed, and the integrity they upheld.

In a crescendo of emotions, the doctor's words reverberated through the air, carrying with them a symphony of joy and relief. "It's a baby boy, and both baby and mother are well," the announcement echoed, igniting a flame of elation within the hearts of Mr. and Mrs. Sharma. Tears of sheer happiness welled up in their eyes, shimmering like diamonds in the sunlight. At that moment, time seemed to stand still as they embraced the profound miracle that had unfolded before them. Their hearts overflowed with indescribable love as their precious son entered the world, a testament to their shared journey and unwavering devotion.

In the arms of the doctor, their little bundle of joy lay, fragile yet resilient, a perfect reflection of the love that had created him. As Mr. Sharma gazed upon his newborn son, a surge of emotions engulfed him, blending awe, gratitude, and an overwhelming sense of responsibility. The weight of this newfound love, as it settled upon their shoulders! Their hearts swelled with a love so profound it transcended the boundaries of their beings. In that tiny, fragile life, they saw the embodiment of their hopes, dreams, and endless possibilities. Every beat of his heart harmonized with theirs, forming an unbreakable bond that would guide them through the journey of parenthood.

As their son was placed in Mrs. Sharma's arms, a surge of tenderness washed over her. The sheer magnitude of this moment brought tears of joy streaming down her cheeks. In that instant, the world around them seemed to fade away, leaving only the blissful embrace of mother and child.

Family 2

The legacy of the textile business was passed down from generation to generation, from father to son. When Mr. Patel took over the reins from his beloved father, he felt a mix of emotions swirling within him—excitement, gratitude, and a tinge of nervousness. The weight of the responsibility he now carried on his shoulders was both exhilarating and daunting. As he stepped into his new role, memories flooded his mind, reminding him of the countless hours he spent by his father's side, learning the intricacies of the textile industry. The scent of freshly woven fabrics, the rhythmic hum of the machines, and the bustling energy of the factory floor all evoked a deep sense of nostalgia.

The path ahead was not without challenges. The textile industry had its ups and downs, and Mr. Patel was aware of the fierce competition that awaited him. Yet, he was determined to honor his father's hard work and dedication. Every thread woven by his father represented not just a product but a piece of their family's history and the dreams they nurtured together. With each passing day, Mr. Patel poured his heart and soul into the business. He meticulously nurtured the relationships his father had built with suppliers, ensuring the continued availability of the finest raw materials. He embraced innovation and technology, introducing modern machinery and processes to streamline operations without compromising the craftsmanship his father had instilled in him.

There were moments of doubt when challenges seemed insurmountable and the weight of expectations threatened to overwhelm him. But he drew strength from the lessons his father taught him—the importance of perseverance, integrity, and staying true to his values. He knew that success would require not just hard work but also resilience and a willingness to adapt to changing times. And so, Mr. Patel persevered. He kept the flame of his father's legacy alive, breathing new life into the textile business. Slowly but surely, his efforts began to bear fruit. Customers appreciated the quality of his products and the attention to detail that permeated every stitch. Orders poured in, and the business flourished under his guidance.

As Mr. Patel advanced in his career, an unexpected turn of events awaited him. His father, deeply invested in his son's happiness and the prosperity of the business, made a decision that stirred a whirlwind of emotions within Mr. Patel's heart. He proposed an alliance that went beyond business—an alliance of hearts and minds. The prospect of marriage, intertwined with the textile business, seemed both exciting and uncertain to Mr. Patel. His father, in his wisdom, had chosen a partner who possessed not only beauty but also a wealth of knowledge and education. The daughter of their business partner, she was a symbol of refinement and sophistication.

Mr. Patel couldn't help but feel a mixture of curiosity and trepidation as he contemplated this new chapter in his life. Would their union strengthen the bonds between the families and fortify the business further? Or would it add unexpected complexities to the delicate balance he had strived so hard to achieve? As he met the young lady for the first time, he was struck by her grace and intelligence. Conversations flowed effortlessly, revealing shared aspirations and values. She spoke with a passion for the textile industry, her eyes sparkling with an understanding of its intricate nuances. It was clear that she, too, held a deep reverence for the business that had become an inseparable part of their lives.

In the days that followed, Mr. Patel found himself captivated by her presence. Their shared dreams and visions for the future ignited a spark within him, fanning the flames of possibility. Their discussions ventured beyond mere transactions and profits; they delved into the artistry of textiles, the impact they could make in the world, and the legacy they were destined to leave behind. As he sought solace in the comforting presence of his father, he realized the wisdom embedded in his father's choice. Their union would not only unite two families but also create a formidable partnership grounded in mutual respect and shared goals. The young lady's education and insight would bring fresh perspectives to the business, infusing it with innovation and a broader understanding of the global market.

With each passing day, Mr. Patel's heart embraced the idea of this union. The prospect of a life intertwined with his business partner's daughter grew from an uncertain notion into a beacon of hope. Their marriage would not only enrich their personal lives but also propel the textile business to new heights, with their combined strengths propelling them forward. And so, as he stood at the precipice of this new chapter, Mr. Patel felt gratitude for his father's wisdom and the love that guided his choices. He knew that the path ahead would be one of discovery and growth, where love and business would dance in perfect harmony. And with a heart full of anticipation, he eagerly awaited the day when he would embark on this new adventure, hand in hand with his soon-to-be wife, ready to embrace the joys and challenges that lay before them.

At the age of 30, Mr. Patel found himself entering into a sacred union bound by love and tradition. His path crossed with that of an educated young woman, hailing from a family deeply rooted in the world of business. It was an arranged marriage, a union of two souls destined to walk hand in hand, embarking on a journey filled with shared dreams and aspirations. As Mr. Patel laid his eyes upon his bride for the first time, a wave of joy and anticipation washed over him. Her radiant smile, a reflection of her inner beauty, captivated his heart. In her eyes, he saw a kindred spirit, someone who understood the essence of their joint family's legacy.

From the very beginning, their love blossomed amidst the bustling corridors of the textile business. Together, they wove a tapestry of mutual respect and admiration, blending their individual strengths to form an unbreakable bond. Mr. Patel, with his liberal mindset, embraced his wife's ambitions wholeheartedly, knowing that her aspirations were as valuable as his own. Side by side, they faced the challenges that life and business threw their way. Their decisions, crafted with wisdom and foresight, bore the mark of a harmonious partnership. Whether it was expanding their business horizons or nurturing their growing family, they approached each choice as a united front, their love serving as a guiding light.

The strength of their relationship lay in their unwavering support for one another. Mr. Patel celebrated his wife's accomplishments with an overflowing heart, rejoicing in her triumphs as if they were his own. In turn, his wife stood by his side, offering encouragement and lending her sharp intellect to the growth of the business. Their love was not confined to the confines of the boardroom or the walls of their home. It transcended boundaries and embraced the beauty of life itself. Together, they embarked on adventures, creating memories that would forever be etched in their hearts. Whether it was sharing laughter under a starlit sky or finding solace in each other's arms during trying times, their love was a sanctuary, a refuge from the storms of life.

As Mrs. Patel sat in the business meeting, the room filled with the hum of conversations and the weight of important decisions. Amidst the professional setting, a beautiful secret nestled within her heart, waiting to be shared with her beloved husband. A rush of emotions overwhelmed her as she realized she was carrying the most precious gift of all—a tiny life growing within her. With anticipation coursing through her veins, Mrs. Patel couldn't contain her joy any longer. She longed to embrace her husband, to whisper the magical news into his ear and watch his eyes light up with a mix of surprise and delight. And so, she carefully crafted a romantic date, a moment in time when their love would intertwine with the sheer wonder of new life.

As the evening unfolded, Mrs. Patel's heart danced with a mix of nervousness and sheer excitement. The soft glow of candlelight illuminated the room, casting a warm and intimate ambiance. Their eyes met, filled with a love that had weathered storms and celebrated victories together. With trembling hands, Mrs. Patel took hold of her husband's, feeling the familiar touch that always brought her solace. She gazed into his eyes, finding solace in the depths of his unwavering love. In that sacred moment, she shared the news that would forever change their lives.

As the words slipped from her lips, a radiant smile graced Mrs. Patel's face. The room seemed to hold its breath, suspended in the weight of their shared joy. Time stood still as her husband's eyes widened, mirroring the elation that filled her own heart. It was a moment of pure magic, a celebration of the love that had created a new life within her. Throughout the entirety of Mrs. Patel's pregnancy, her husband, Mr. Patel, spared no expense in ensuring that she received the utmost care and comfort. Every step of the way, he stood as her unwavering support, embracing the responsibility of providing her with the best facilities and services that money could offer.

From the very first fluttering kicks that stirred within Mrs. Patel's womb to the momentous day of their child's birth, every memory etched itself into the fabric of their lives. Mr. Patel spared no effort in making this journey an extraordinary one, a testament to his unyielding love and devotion. As the time drew near for their child to enter the world, Mr. Patel meticulously researched and chose the most reputable and luxurious hospital where the finest medical professionals would be at hand. He ensured that no expense was spared in creating a haven of care where Mrs. Patel could feel safe and cherished as she brought their precious child into the world.

In the hallowed halls of that remarkable hospital, Mrs. Patel's every need was met with the utmost attention. The air was permeated with a sense of serenity and hope, reassuring her that this momentous occasion would be nothing short of extraordinary. Skilled doctors and nurses enveloped her with compassion, providing round-the-clock care, their expertise serving as a beacon of reassurance amidst the beautiful chaos of childbirth. The ninth month of Mrs. Patel's pregnancy had arrived, filling the air with a mixture of excitement and anticipation. The couple eagerly awaited the arrival of their little bundle of joy, dreaming of the joyous moments they would share as a family. But fate had a different plan in store—one that would test their strength and resilience.

As the day of Mrs. Patel's delivery approached, Mr. Patel found himself torn between his responsibilities. A crucial business meeting called him away, a meeting he couldn't simply postpone. Every fiber of his being resisted leaving his beloved wife's side during such a significant moment, but duty compelled him to board that flight. The separation was agonizing for both Mr. and Mrs. Patel. As the plane soared higher into the sky, Mr. Patel's heart remained grounded with his wife, entwined in the bittersweet emotions of longing and helplessness. He yearned to be there to hold her hand and to provide the support she deserved during this transformative experience.

Meanwhile, in the hospital, Mrs. Patel clung to her strength, surrounded by her loving family. Each contraction intensified the pain and longing she felt for her husband. She yearned for his comforting presence, the reassurance of his touch, and the shared experience of welcoming their child together. The absence of his familiar face cast a shadow over the room, amplifying the intensity of the moment.

And then, as if the universe conspired to weave a tale of resilience and love, the baby boy arrived—the room filled with joyous cries, mingling with tears of both happiness and longing. The little one's first breaths echoed through the walls, intertwining with Mrs. Patel's and resonating with the unspoken bond between mother and child. In the midst of this emotional rollercoaster, Mr. Patel raced against time, propelled by a fierce determination to join his family. Every passing second felt like an eternity as he journeyed back to his wife and the child he had yet to hold. The weight of guilt and regret threatened to overwhelm him, but his unwavering love for his family carried him forward.

Finally, the moment arrived. With trembling hands and a heart bursting with emotions, Mr. Patel stepped into the hospital room. The love in his eyes mirrored the intensity of the journey he had just undertaken. As he held his newborn son for the first time, a profound sense of awe washed over him. The tiny fingers curled around his own as if acknowledging their unbreakable connection. Tears welled up in Mr. Patel's eyes as he embraced his wife, his soul entwined with hers in an embrace that transcended words. The birth of their child became a testament to their love, their unwavering commitment to one another and their family. It was a bittersweet reminder that even in the face of separation, love could triumph, bridging the distance and binding them together.

Family 3

Mr. Singh was born into a middle-class family with great aspirations. He possessed an unwavering determination to make his dreams a reality. As a diligent student, he consistently displayed obedience and dedication to his studies. Eventually, his hard work paid off, and he managed to secure a respectable, well-paying job. Mr. Singh's journey was marked by his relentless pursuit of his goals. He remained focused and undeterred, leaving no stone unturned in his quest for success. Despite the challenges he encountered along the way, he never wavered in his determination to achieve his ambitions. His educational background laid a strong foundation for his career. Armed with knowledge and a thirst for growth, Mr. Singh embraced the opportunities that came his way as India expanded its global presence. He understood the significance of this transformative period and was determined to capitalize on it.

The new job that Mr. Singh undertook was indeed challenging, but it sparked a sense of excitement within him. He embraced the difficulties that came with it, viewing them as opportunities for growth and development. As time passed, Mr. Singh's dedication and hard work propelled him to become the top-performing employee in the corporate world. The challenges of his role did not deter Mr. Singh; instead, they ignited his passion and drove to excel. He approached his work with enthusiasm and a commitment to continuous improvement. Through his perseverance and a hunger for success, he quickly gained recognition for his exceptional performance.

Colleagues and superiors alike began to acknowledge Mr. Singh's outstanding abilities and contributions. His consistent commitment to excellence set him apart from others in the corporate realm. With each achievement, he raised the bar higher and set new standards for himself. Mr.

Singh's ascent to becoming the best-performing employee in the corporate world was a testament to his unwavering work ethic and determination. His success was not a stroke of luck but the result of his relentless pursuit of excellence. He continually sought new challenges, eagerly taking on responsibilities that pushed his limits and broadened his skill set.

As Mr. Singh's accomplishments piled up, his reputation soared. He became a source of inspiration and a role model for his colleagues. Many sought his guidance and aspired to emulate his work ethic and success. His journey served as a reminder that dedication, resilience, and a thirst for growth are key ingredients for achieving remarkable feats in the corporate world.

As Mr. Singh continued to excel in his career, he found himself developing romantic feelings for his colleague, Taniya, who shared his desire for independence. Their personalities complemented each other, and their shared mindset brought them closer together. Eventually, they made the heartfelt decision to marry each other. Their love blossomed amidst their shared ambitions and aspirations. Both Mr. Singh and Mrs. Singh understood the importance of personal growth and supporting each other's dreams. They saw in each other a partner who would encourage and empower them to pursue their individual goals while building a life together.

Their decision to marry was not only based on love but also on a deep understanding and respect for each other's independence and aspirations. They recognized the value of a partnership built on shared values and a shared vision for the future. As they embarked on their journey as a married couple, Mr. Singh and Mrs. Singh continued to support and uplift each other. They celebrated each other's achievements, providing unwavering encouragement and a strong foundation for personal and professional growth.

Mr. Singh and his spouse became a source of inspiration for others, demonstrating that love and ambition can coexist harmoniously. They showed that a supportive and understanding partner could fuel personal and professional success, fostering an environment where both individuals can pursue their dreams while nurturing a loving relationship. Together, Mr. Singh and his spouse embraced their shared journey, celebrating their independence and cherishing the bond they had formed. They stood as a testament to the belief that true love not only supports personal growth but also strengthens the pursuit of individual dreams, creating a life of fulfillment and happiness.

As a working couple, Mr. Singh and Mrs. Singh believed in sharing household responsibilities equally. They understood the importance of maintaining a balanced partnership, where both partners contributed to both their professional and personal lives. As they continued to grow financially independent, they made the heartfelt decision to start a family and have a baby. Knowing that having a child would require adjustments in their lives, Mr. Singh assured Mrs. Singh that she could take a career break without it being the end of her professional journey. He wholeheartedly supported her decision and reassured her that she would have the opportunity to resume her job after a year.

As Mr. Singh and Mrs. Singh had entered into a love marriage, there was initially a sense of dissatisfaction among some family members. However, as time went on, the news of Taniya's pregnancy brought immense joy and happiness to both of their families. The arrival of their baby boy was seen as a blessing that helped bridge the gap and rebuild the relationships between the couple and their parents. The joyous news of Taniya's pregnancy brought about a transformation within the families. The impending arrival of a new life created an atmosphere of love, unity, and togetherness. Both Mr. Singh and Taniya's parents were overjoyed to welcome their grandchild into the world, and their hearts swelled with affection and happiness.

The birth of their baby boy became a turning point in the family dynamics. It served as a reminder of the unconditional love that existed within the bonds of family, helping to dissolve any lingering dissatisfaction and bringing everyone closer. The couple's parents recognized the immense joy and fulfillment that their grandchild would bring to their lives, and they eagerly embraced the new chapter that was unfolding before them. The arrival of the baby also provided an opportunity for Mr. Singh and Mrs. Singh to strengthen their bond with their own parents. The couple welcomed the support and guidance offered by their families during this precious time, and the shared experience of welcoming a new member into the family created a profound sense of connection and understanding.

Through the gift of their baby, Mr. Singh and Mrs. Singh were able to mend any strained relationships and regain the love and acceptance of their parents. The little one became a beacon of love, bringing generations together and fostering an environment of harmony and joy. The experience of becoming parents allowed Mr. Singh and Mrs. Singh to appreciate the value of family even more deeply. It reminded them of the importance of nurturing relationships and cherishing the bonds that connect them to their loved ones. Their journey of parenthood catalyzed healing and rebuilding, strengthening the foundation of their extended family.

During Mrs. Singh's career break, Mr. Singh stepped up to take on additional responsibilities at home, ensuring a nurturing and supportive environment for their growing family. He understood the importance of allowing Mrs. Singh the time and space she needed to bond with their child and adjust to the demands of motherhood. Throughout this period, Mr. Singh remained steadfast in his belief that Taniya's career was an integral part of her identity and personal growth. He provided continuous encouragement, assuring her that her professional aspirations were valid and would be waiting for her when she decided to return to work.

Takeaways:

- ★ Reflect on the transformative power of education.
- ★ Embrace resilience in the face of challenges.
- ★ Cherish and support your partner in the journey of life.
- ★ Embrace challenges in business with innovation and resilience.
- ★ Recognize the value of alliances that go beyond business, fostering mutual respect and shared goals.
- ★ Appreciate the harmonious integration of personal and professional life, understanding that love can enhance and not hinder success.
- ★ Embrace challenges as opportunities for growth and development.
- ★ Recognize the value of a partnership built on shared values and a shared vision for the future.
- ★ Celebrate personal and professional achievements within a supportive and understanding relationship.
- ★ Understand and appreciate the importance of family bonds and the transformative power of parenthood.

Shades of Life

Chapter 2

Shades of Character

"In the grand narrative of existence, our lives are painted in the rich and vibrant hues of diverse experiences, forging the unique and intricate masterpiece that is the mosaic of our individual shades of character."

Family 1

Mr. and Mrs. Sharma carefully chose the name Vinay for their baby boy, knowing that it symbolized important qualities such as guidance, good behavior, genuineness, politeness, modesty, and smartness. They had high aspirations for their son, driven by the hardships Mr. Sharma had experienced in his own life. Determined to shield Vinay from similar struggles, they nevertheless desired to impart upon him a deep understanding of life's realities. Above all, Mr. Sharma wished Vinay to develop unwavering ethical and moral strength, even in adversity. He understood that life could present challenges and wanted his son to possess the resilience and integrity necessary to navigate difficult times with grace. From a young age, Mr. and Mrs. Sharma instilled in Vinay the importance of treating others with respect and kindness. They emphasized the value of honesty and taught him the significance of staying true to oneself, no matter the circumstances. They encouraged him to be modest and humble, never letting success or achievements overshadow his genuine character.

Furthermore, they fostered Vinay's intellectual growth and encouraged him to be a lifelong learner. They believed that knowledge would empower him to make informed decisions and navigate life's complexities with wisdom. They exposed him to various perspectives and encouraged critical thinking, preparing him to confront the challenges that lay ahead. Throughout his upbringing, Vinay witnessed his parents' own commitment to these principles. Mr. Sharma shared stories of his own struggles, demonstrating the importance of perseverance and determination. He imparted valuable life lessons, illustrating the power of resilience and the significance of maintaining one's integrity even when faced with difficult choices.

Mrs. Sharma, in addition to Mr. Sharma, played a vital role in shaping Vinay's character and instilling in him the values of truthfulness and hard work. She often drew examples from the ancient Indian epics, the Ramayana and the Mahabharata, to emphasize the importance of honesty in every aspect of life. Vinay imbibed these teachings and understood that being truthful was the solution to many challenges one may face. Mrs. Sharma also emphasized the significance of hard work and the pursuit of knowledge as tools to strengthen one's life. She believed Vinay could overcome obstacles and achieve greatness through dedication and continuous learning. At the tender age of six, Vinay had absorbed the sacred stories of the epics, reciting them effortlessly from memory. His profound understanding of these narratives was evident to all who interacted with him, leaving no doubt that he was indeed the son of a knowledgeable and inspiring teacher. Vinay's identity as a teacher's son was unmistakable. His character reflected the values and teachings instilled in him by his parents. Through the stories of the epics, coupled with their own exemplary behavior, Mr. and Mrs. Sharma had nurtured in Vinay a strong moral compass and a deep appreciation for the power of truthfulness and hard work.

One day, Mrs. Sharma took Vinay along with her to the market to buy groceries. As they strolled through the bustling aisles, Vinay's eyes caught sight of a tempting chocolate display. He longed to savor the sweet treat but noticed that his mother had only brought enough money for their essential purchases. Respectfully, he kept his desire to himself and refrained from asking for the chocolate. As they completed their shopping and headed towards the exit, the last vendor accidentally dropped a 10/- note. Vinay could have easily kept the money and fulfilled his wish for the chocolate, but his inherent honesty guided him. Without hesitation, he turned back and approached the vendor.

In a soft voice, Vinay said, "Uncle, you dropped the money by mistake." Surprised by the young boy's integrity, the vendor smiled warmly and thanked Vinay for his honesty. Touched by Vinay's act of integrity, the vendor offered him toffee as a small reward for his honesty. However, Vinay graciously declined the offer, politely saying, "Uncle, I have only done what is right. It's nothing extraordinary. I will surely buy from you when I bring my own money next time."

Mrs. Sharma couldn't help but feel a surge of pride and admiration for her young son. His maturity and understanding at such a tender age brought tears of joy to her eyes. She hugged Vinay tightly, expressing her pride in his moral character. This incident left a lasting impact on Vinay. It reinforced the importance of honesty, even when faced with the temptation to benefit oneself. Vinay understood that doing the right thing brought a sense of inner fulfillment and maintained the trust and respect of others.

When Mr. Sharma returned home and learned about the incident, he was deeply moved by Vinay's unwavering honesty. Filled with pride and admiration, he immediately headed to the nearby shop and purchased a big chocolate for his son. As Mr. Sharma presented the chocolate to Vinay, he lovingly said, "Son, your integrity and truthfulness deserve a reward. Remember, the rewards of honesty and truthfulness are always bigger than any immediate gratification." Vinay listened attentively to his father's words, taking in the profound lesson embedded within.

At that moment, Vinay realized the deeper meaning behind his decision to return the extra money. He understood that if he had succumbed to his desire for the toffee, he would have missed out on the greater reward—both the joy of doing what was right and the larger chocolate his father had bought for him. With a sense of contentment and appreciation, Vinay embraced his father's wisdom. He understood that honesty and truthfulness were not merely about avoiding punishment or seeking rewards but about upholding one's values and maintaining personal integrity. Vinay realized that the true measure of a person's character lies in their ability to make ethical choices, even when faced with temptation.

From that day forward, Vinay carried this valuable lesson with him. The incident not only deepened his understanding of honesty but also reinforced his belief in the intrinsic rewards that come from doing what is right. He cherished the big chocolate as a symbol of the greater rewards that awaited him whenever he chose integrity over immediate gratification. Mr. Sharma's thoughtful gesture and wise words further strengthened the bond between father and son. Their shared understanding of the importance of honesty and the enduring value of integrity created a lifelong connection grounded in mutual respect and admiration. Vinay's experience constantly reminded him that the rewards of honesty extend beyond material possessions. They encompass self-respect, trust, and the knowledge that one's actions positively impact the world.

The incident became a cherished memory for the Sharma family, a testament to the power of honesty, and a reminder of the lasting rewards that come from doing what is right.

As the time for Vinay's school admission approached, Mr. Sharma meticulously planned for his son's future. He researched various schools in the city, seeking an institution that would provide Vinay with an excellent education and a nurturing environment. Among the options, Mumbai's 'City School' stood out, renowned for its commitment to excellence and its proximity to its house. Mr. Sharma considered all aspects, weighing the quality of education, extracurricular activities, and the school's overall reputation. He was determined that Vinay's access to quality education would not be hindered by any financial constraints.

With steadfast resolve, Mr. Sharma made the decision to enroll Vinay at Mumbai's City School, believing that it would provide him with the best opportunities for growth and learning. He was determined to ensure that Vinay received every advantage possible to shape his future and overcome the challenges Mr. Sharma had faced in his own life. He made the necessary arrangements and completed the admission process for Vinay. The excitement filled the air as they prepared for the new chapter in Vinay's educational journey.

Family 2

The atmosphere at the naming ceremony was vibrant and filled with excitement. The venue was adorned with colorful decorations, reflecting the joyful mood of the gathering. Guests arrived dressed in their finest attire, ready to share in the Patel family's happiness and celebrate the arrival of little Vaibhav. As the ceremony commenced, the family stood together, beaming with pride as they introduced their son to the world. The name Vaibhav, chosen for their son, holds the meaning of "grand," symbolizing the bright and prosperous future they envision for him. The celebration was a joyous occasion filled with love, blessings, and a spirit of giving, reflecting the Patel family's values and their desire to create a positive impact in the world around them.

Mrs. Patel held baby Vaibhav gently in her arms while Mr. Patel stood beside her, his face radiant with paternal joy. They expressed their gratitude to everyone present, acknowledging the significance of their loved one's presence in their lives. In a heartfelt speech, Mr. Patel spoke of the hopes and dreams he and his wife held for their son. He emphasized the importance of love, education, and compassion, vowing to provide Vaibhav with every opportunity to grow and succeed. The room resonated with heartfelt applause and words of encouragement from the guests, offering their support and blessings to the young boy.

Following the formalities, the celebration continued with delicious food and lively music. The aroma of mouthwatering dishes filled the air as everyone indulged in a sumptuous feast. Laughter and conversations echoed throughout the venue as guests shared stories, reminisced about fond memories, and expressed their good wishes for the future of little Vaibhav. Amidst the revelry, the Patels ensured that their celebration also carried a deeper purpose. They organized a charitable initiative where they distributed food and provided financial assistance to those in need. Their generous act of giving exemplified their commitment to instilling compassion and empathy in their son's upbringing, teaching him the importance of supporting others and giving back to the community.

As the day drew to a close, the Patels expressed their gratitude once again, extending heartfelt thanks to all who had graced the occasion with their presence. The naming ceremony of Vaibhav had been a resounding success, not only as a celebration of his arrival but also as an expression of the Patel family's unity, love, and dedication to making a positive difference in the world. With their hearts full of love and hope, the Patels looked forward to the journey of parenthood, guided by the meaning of their son's name, Vaibhav, reminding them of the grand possibilities that lay ahead. The celebration had left an indelible mark on their lives, forever etching the joyous beginning of their son's life in their hearts and the hearts of all who had shared in the occasion.

Vaibhav's childhood was indeed privileged, surrounded by luxuries and a loving family. During the day, he would often spend time with his doting grandparents, who showered him with affection and wisdom. Despite their busy schedules, his parents made a conscious effort to allocate quality time to be with their son, recognizing the importance of nurturing their bond and being present in his life.

As Vaibhav grew older, he became increasingly aware of the fortunate circumstances he was born into. He witnessed firsthand the success and growth of his family's business, which seemed to flourish alongside his arrival. The prosperity that accompanied his presence served as a reminder of the blessings and opportunities he enjoyed.

Shades of Life

Despite growing up in a life of luxury, Vaibhav possessed an unwavering spirit that refused to accept defeat. His determination to achieve the best permeated every aspect of his being. On this particular day, while engaged in play with his neighboring friends, the children collectively decided to partake in a race. News of the race reached Mr. Patel, who, eager to motivate the children, promised to reward the winner with new clothes. Filled with anticipation, the children swiftly made their way to the nearby playground, with Vaibhav leading the charge and reaching the destination first.

Vaibhav, having been accustomed to a comfortable lifestyle, carried a slightly heavier build, which might have seemingly diminished his chances of winning a race against more physically fit opponents. However, this did not deter his enthusiasm in the slightest. With determination gleaming in his eyes, he stood poised at the starting line, ready to give his all and prove that appearances could be deceiving.

The race commenced, and baby Vaibhav exerted all his strength, determined to run faster than ever before. However, despite his best efforts, he found himself trailing behind one of the participants. Vaibhav was on the verge of securing second place when the child ahead suddenly stopped, crying out in pain. A thorn had pierced his leg, and the running track was strewn with minor stones that had hindered the other children.

In an unexpected turn of events, Vaibhav found himself winning the race. Although he felt a sense of happiness and accomplishment, a twinge of suspicion lingered within the nanny and the other mothers. It seemed unfair that the other children had been unable to run smoothly due to the presence of obstacles. It was a matter of luck that Vaibhav had emerged victorious. Mr. Patel observed his son's behavior during the race and felt a hint of confusion. He wondered why Vaibhav had chosen a specific running track and stood determinedly at that spot. It appeared as though he had noticed the hurdles and strategically selected the best possible track. Although he could only assume, Mr. Patel believed that Vaibhav's keen observation had influenced his decision, allowing him to navigate the race more effectively.

In the evening, Vaibhav excitedly approached his grandfather & mother, showcasing the prize he had won from the race. Mr. Patel's face brightened with happiness as he celebrated his grandson's victory. However, his father chimed in, informing the parents about the injuries sustained by the other children during the race. Concern was etched across his face. To their surprise, Vaibhav wore a knowing smile as if he possessed a deeper understanding of the situation. His parents observed his expression, puzzled yet curious. In response, Mr. Patel reassured his son, acknowledging that accidents and injuries were common occurrences in children's races. He expressed pride in Vaibhav's achievement, emphasizing that winning the race was remarkable.

Drawing upon an analogy, Mr. Patel shared a perspective with Vaibhav the next day. He likened life's challenges to a rainstorm, where different people choose varied ways to navigate through it. Some opt for umbrellas, others don raincoats, and some simply walk in the rain. Ultimately, what truly matters is reaching the destination, irrespective of the chosen method. Vaibhav absorbed his father's words, contemplating their significance. He realized that winning was indeed a crucial aspect of life. It represented the culmination of efforts, perseverance, and determination. While the injuries suffered by the other children were unfortunate, they didn't diminish the value of Vaibhav's victory. It was a moment to be celebrated and cherished. The conversation with his father instilled in Vaibhav a profound understanding—that in life, success should be embraced and celebrated, regardless of the circumstances surrounding it. It was a lesson that winning held its own significance, independent of the experiences of others.

In the days following, Vaibhav's parents made the decision to enroll him in Mumbai's City School. They believed that providing him with a quality education would pave the way for a bright and successful future. Mumbai's City School was renowned for its academic excellence, comprehensive curriculum, and nurturing environment. Vaibhav's first day at the new school was filled with a mix of excitement and nervousness. As he stepped through the school gates, he was greeted by a vibrant atmosphere buzzing with the energy of students engaged in various activities. The campus was sprawling, adorned with colorful classrooms, playgrounds, and learning centers. Vaibhav's parents accompanied him, ensuring a smooth transition into his new educational journey. They met with the school staff, who warmly welcomed them and provided them with all the necessary information and guidance. The caring and supportive environment of the school reassured Vaibhav's parents that they had made the right choice.

Family 3

The Singh family had meticulously planned a naming ceremony for their newborn, while Mr. Singh tirelessly dedicated himself to a crucial project. He was acutely aware that successfully cracking the client would unlock a world of opportunities, including a significant appraisal and the possibility of a well-deserved promotion. As guests started arriving at their houses on this auspicious day, anticipation filled the air, shared equally by the parents and the visitors. The baby was being prepared for the momentous occasion, and just as the time to choose a name approached, Mr. Singh's boss made an unexpected announcement that reverberated through the room. With a broad smile, he revealed that Mr. Singh had indeed secured the client, instantly turning the day into a celebration of double joy. The news spread like wildfire, engulfing the atmosphere with excitement and elation. A wave of congratulatory wishes flooded in from family members, friends, and colleagues, who were all thrilled to be part of this extraordinary achievement. The revelation kindled an electric atmosphere as everyone grasped the significance of this triumph. They understood that destiny had intertwined this joyous event with Mr. Singh's professional success, making the occasion all the more exceptional.

Gratefulness and pride illuminated Mr. Singh's face as he received warm embraces and heartfelt applause. His boss approached him, extending a firm handshake and sincere congratulations, recognizing his exceptional efforts and unwavering determination. The boss emphasized that this outstanding accomplishment would undoubtedly propel Mr. Singh's career to new heights, affirming his worth within the organization. At that moment, Mr. Singh couldn't help but reflect on the countless hours he had poured into his work, the sleepless nights, and the relentless dedication. It was a journey filled with challenges and sacrifices, but this achievement validated every ounce of effort he had invested. He acknowledged the unwavering support of his wife, whose love and understanding had fueled his drive and ambition.

Amidst the joyous atmosphere, the naming ceremony proceeded with an air of jubilation. The gathering resonated with laughter, vibrant conversations, and heartfelt blessings for the newborn. Family and friends gathered around the little one, offering their suggestions for names imbued with meaning and aspirations for a bright future. In that moment of joy and triumph, Mr. Singh made a heartfelt decision. Inspired by the significance of the occasion and the hope for his son's future, he chose to name his newborn son Vijay. The name Vijay, meaning "victory" in Hindi, held deep symbolism and aspirations for the child. Mr. Singh envisioned his son growing up to conquer challenges, achieve great success, and overcome obstacles with determination and resilience. It was a name chosen with love, hope, and an unwavering belief in the extraordinary potential of his beloved child.

The celebration reached its zenith as glasses were raised in a toast to the baby's future and Mr. Singh's continued success. It was a day etched in their memories, a testament to the power of hard work, perseverance, and the unforeseen blessings that life can bestow. The fusion of a joyous naming ceremony with the elation of professional triumph exemplified the magic that can unfold when dedication meets opportunity. As the day drew to a close, the Singh family and their guests departed, carrying with them the indelible memories of this extraordinary occasion. In their hearts, they knew that the convergence of celebration and achievement had marked the beginning of a new chapter, brimming with possibilities and the promise of a brighter future.

Following that momentous day, Mr. Singh shouldered increased responsibilities at home and in the office. His professional commitments grew significantly with his promotion to the position of Chief Regional Head of Kapoor Industries, overseeing financial assistance and investments. Amidst this crucial period, Mr. Singh's wife became his unwavering support pillar, ensuring he didn't miss out on any tasks or opportunities at the office. Together, the couple worked in tandem, striking a delicate balance between their personal and professional lives. Knowing the importance of maintaining a harmonious family life, they made arrangements for a nanny to care for baby Vijay during the day while they were occupied with work. It was essential to them that their little one received the love, care, and attention he deserved, even in their absence.

However, each evening, after a fulfilling day's work, the Singh family cherished their post-dinner moments. It was during this precious time that baby Vijay received undivided attention from his adoring parents. They devoted themselves fully to him, reveling in his innocent laughter, cuddles, and milestones. It was a time for the family to bond, create lasting memories, and strengthen the unbreakable bond between parents and child.

Amidst the abundance and material comforts, Vijay also developed a keen sense of social responsibility. Vijay's parents, recognizing their son's burgeoning awareness and empathy, encouraged his involvement in charitable endeavors. They took him along on visits to orphanages, community service projects, and fundraisers, exposing him to different aspects of philanthropy. These experiences instilled in Vijay a profound understanding of the importance of compassion and the impact one can have on the lives of those less fortunate.

The dedicated nanny, as part of her responsibilities, would often take baby Vijay to the park to engage with other children. She made sure to keep Mr. Singh and his wife updated on Vijay's day-to-day growth, behavior, and activities. During these outings, Vijay couldn't help but notice other children accompanied by their mothers enjoying quality time together, but he did not complain, he was often a silent and understanding child.

Among all the members of the family, there was one special member who shared an extraordinary bond with Vijay - their beloved pet dog. From the moment Vijay came into the world, the dog had been a constant presence, almost like a sibling to him. This close companionship played a significant role in shaping Vijay's affectionate nature towards animals, instilling in him a deep love and respect for all creatures.

As Vijay grew older, his father often pondered what career path would be most suitable for his compassionate and empathetic son. One day, as Vijay played in the garden, he noticed a boy just a few years older than him diligently watering the plants. Intrigued by this young gardener, Vijay approached him with open curiosity and a friendly smile. The two youngsters adjoined hands and struck up a conversation, quickly forming a heartfelt connection.

When Vijay returned from the garden, his father, impressed by his son's interaction with the servant boy, questioned him about what led him to initiate the conversation. Vijay responded with innocence and wisdom beyond his years, saying, "Dad, I noticed that the boy seemed a bit bored, and I saw that he missed watering some plants. When I went to talk to him, not only did he feel happier, but together we were able to water all the plants correctly." Vijay's answer showcased his keen observation skills, empathy, and understanding of human emotions. His ability to perceive the situation and take the initiative to make it better spoke volumes about his intelligence and compassionate nature.

His father listened attentively, realizing that this incident held a profound significance. It provided him with the answer he had been seeking, confirming that Vijay possessed the qualities of a suitable leader. Not only was he compassionate, but he also had the innate ability to inspire and motivate others to achieve a common goal without pressuring or imposing upon them. The incident served as a clear indication that Vijay possessed the qualities necessary to lead with empathy, understanding, and the ability to bring people together. His natural talent for recognizing and addressing the needs of others would undoubtedly make him an exceptional leader in the future.

Recognizing his son's down-to-earth nature and wanting to preserve those qualities, Mr. Singh made a thoughtful decision regarding Vijay's education. He enrolled him in Mumbai's esteemed City School, known for its excellent reputation in providing a well-rounded education. Mr. Singh, aware of the privileges his son enjoyed, requested the teaching staff to treat Vijay as an equal among his peers, encouraging him to forge friendships with all the children. Despite his privileged background, the request to treat Vijay on equal terms reflected Mr. Singh's desire to ensure his son remained grounded and connected with others. By fostering an inclusive environment and encouraging Vijay to interact with children from diverse backgrounds, Mr. Singh believed his son would develop a broader perspective, empathy, and a genuine understanding of people's lives beyond his own.

Takeaways:

★ Instill a strong moral compass and a deep appreciation for truthfulness and hard work from a young age.

★ Stress the importance of quality time in parenting, even in privileged environments.

★ Prioritize quality education for children.

★ Ensure a supportive and nurturing environment for a child's educational journey.

★ Expose children to charitable activities and community service.

★ Instill a sense of empathy and responsibility towards the less fortunate.

★ Recognize and nurture leadership qualities in children.

★ Select educational institutions that prioritize a well-rounded and inclusive education.

★ Encourage interactions with peers from diverse backgrounds to broaden perspectives.

Chapter 3

Paths Diverge

"Life often presents us with circumstances that are beyond our control. Acceptance is a crucial aspect of life."

As the first rays of sunlight peeked through the curtains, Vinay, Vaibhav, and Vijay's hearts fluttered with a mix of excitement and nervousness. Today was the first day of school, a day filled with new adventures and discoveries. But stepping out of the comforting embrace of home was no easy task for the younger ones. Curiosity danced in their eyes, eager to explore the unknown corridors and classrooms that awaited them. Thoughts raced through their mind, wondering what their new teacher would be like, what subjects they would learn, and if they would make friends along the way. The world outside seemed vast and mysterious, but the children's yearning for knowledge burned brighter than any fear.

The three children took hesitant steps towards the school gate, their small hands clutching tightly onto their parent's reassuring grasp. The bustling sounds and bustling sights overwhelmed their senses, momentarily intensifying their apprehension. Yet, a glimmer of hope sparkled within, as they spotted other children in uniforms, all sharing similar emotions. As they entered the classroom, their gaze darted around, taking in the vibrant displays and welcoming smiles from their classmates. The once-dreaded fear slowly gave way to anticipation. Each introduction and exchange of names felt like unlocking a new chapter of possibilities.

They discovered the potential for lifelong friendships in that room filled with unfamiliar faces.

Throughout the day, the children's hearts swelled with a mix of awe and excitement. In the bustling school cafeteria, Vinay, Vijay, and Vaibhav found themselves sitting at different tables, each engrossed in their own world, oblivious to one another's presence. It was lunchtime, and as the three boys unfolded their lunch boxes, their meals painted a vivid picture of their distinct preferences.

Vinay's lunch box contained a simple yet comforting meal of daal chawal (lentils and rice). With his hands gently folded, Vinay closed his eyes and silently said a prayer, expressing gratitude for the food before him. His good manners and reverence for mealtime caught Vijay's attention.

Vijay, intrigued by Vinay's prayer, was inspired to strike up a conversation. He approached Vinay's table, his curiosity shining in his eyes. "Hello," Vijay greeted softly. "I noticed you praying before your meal. That's a nice thing to do. Do you always pray before eating?"

Vinay, pleasantly surprised by Vijay's friendly approach, nodded and replied, "Yes, I do. It's a way of showing gratitude for the food we receive. It helps me appreciate the effort that goes into preparing it."

A spark of connection ignited between Vinay and Vijay as they bonded over their shared values and respect for mealtime rituals. Meanwhile, Vaibhav, who had been observing the interaction from his own table, finished his thali, which consisted of rotis, chawal (rice), and a sweet delicacy. Unaware of the other's presence, Vaibhav stood up, about to discard the remaining rotis into the nearby dustbin. However, Vinay and Vijay noticed his action and sprang into action. "Wait!" Vinay called out, rushing toward Vaibhav with a concerned expression. "Don't throw away the rotis. It's not good to waste food."

Vijay quickly joined Vinay's plea, adding, "We should value the food we have. There are many people who don't have enough to eat." Startled by their sudden intervention, Vaibhav hesitated for a moment, his mischievous demeanor fading as he realized the importance of their words. Feeling a sense of guilt, he whispered nervously, "Okay, I won't throw them away. But please don't tell the teachers." Vinay and Vijay, understanding Vaibhav's fear, assured him, "Don't worry, we won't tell anyone. But let's always promise to be mindful of not wasting food." This first brief conversation between the three children planted the seeds of friendship.

As the school bell rang, signaling the end of the day, the three fathers straightened their posture, their eyes fixated on the entrance. And then, in a flurry of laughter and chatter, children burst through the gates, their youthful energy infectious. The fathers' hearts skipped a beat as they spotted their sons among the sea of students. Mr. Sharma's eyes welled up with tears of joy as he saw his son rushing toward him, his arms outstretched for a warm embrace. Mr. Patel's pride swelled as he caught sight of his son, a glimmer of excitement in his eyes, eagerly looking for his father. And Mr. Singh's face lit up with a smile as his son's eyes locked with his, a sense of comfort and security instantly washing over him. In that moment, time seemed to stand still as the fathers enveloped their sons in warm, reassuring hugs. Each embrace conveyed an unspoken message of love, support, and unwavering commitment. The world around them melted away as they listened intently to their sons' animated stories, treasuring every word and cherishing the bond they shared.

In Mr. Sharma's house, the family gathered around the dinner table, eager to hear about the first day of school. As Mr. Sharma listened to his son's animated storytelling, a smile of pride adorned his face. His heart swelled with joy as his son shared how he remembered to pray before lunch and how he had stood up against food wastage by preventing another child from throwing away their food. With a gentle pat on his son's back, Mr. Sharma expressed his happiness, saying, "I'm proud of you, my son. You not only remembered your manners but also showed kindness and responsibility. Remember, it's important to choose friends who share similar values. Keep being wise in your choices and surround yourself with friends who uplift you and encourage good habits."

In Mr. Patel's house, the dinner table was filled with warmth and contentment. Mrs. Patel couldn't help but check her son's lunch box with a beaming smile. To her delight, she found it empty, a clear indication that Vaibhav had enjoyed his meal. Curious, Mrs. Patel asked, "Vaibhav, did you finish your lunch today?" Vaibhav, with a mischievous grin, replied confidently, "Yes, Mom. I am going to school, so I won't miss a chance to learn good manners. In fact, not only did I finish my lunch, but I also made sure to prevent other children from wasting food. I even shared my meal with someone who forgot to bring lunch." Mrs. Patel's heart swelled with pride and joy, knowing that her son was growing up to be a compassionate and considerate young boy. She encouraged him, saying, "That's wonderful, Vaibhav. Keep up the kindness and generosity. Your actions can make a positive impact on others. Always remember to be the best version of yourself."

In Mr. Singh's home, the family gathered around the dinner table, eager to hear Vijay's account of his first day at school. As Vijay enthusiastically narrated the story of his newfound friendship with Vinay, Mr. Singh couldn't contain his happiness. He saw the sparkle in his son's eyes and the genuine joy that radiated from him. Mr. Singh embraced Vijay, expressing his joy, and said, "I'm thrilled to see you making friends, Vijay. True friendships are precious, and it seems like you have found a special one in Vinay. Cherish that friendship and continue to be a good friend yourself. Together, you can learn, grow, and support each other through this wonderful journey of life."

In each household, the parents couldn't help but feel immense pride in their children's actions and choices on their first day of school. They recognized the importance of instilling values such as kindness, responsibility, and wise decision-making. As they continued to nurture and guide their children, they knew that their little ones were on a path toward becoming compassionate, thoughtful individuals who would make a positive impact in the world.

As a couple of years passed, the children continued their journey of learning and growth in school. Vinay remained the epitome of obedience, always following the rules and diligently completing his assignments. His sincerity and respectful demeanor earned him the title of the most obedient child in the class. The teachers appreciated his dedication and held him up as an example for others to follow. Vijay, on the other hand, shone brightly with his intellectual brilliance. His thirst for knowledge and remarkable academic performance made him the favorite of many teachers. With his sharp mind and keen understanding, he effortlessly grasped complex concepts, leaving his classmates in awe. The teachers admired his curiosity and encouraged his pursuit of excellence. As the days went by, Vinay and Vijay's friendship continued to bloom. Their innocent bond grew stronger as they supported and inspired each other. They spent their breaks discussing books, solving puzzles, and exploring the world around them. They formed an unbreakable duo, helping each other navigate the challenges of school life while cherishing their shared experiences.

Meanwhile, Vaibhav remained mischievous, often seeking attention through his pranks and playful antics. He led a circle of friends with his lively and charismatic personality. While he enjoyed being the center of attention, he also recognized the value of spending time with Vinay and Vijay when he needed their support or assistance. They were the ones he turned to when he required guidance or a listening ear. Though their personalities differed, Vinay, Vijay, and Vaibhav had found a unique balance within their friendship. Vinay's obedient nature provided a stable foundation, Vijay's brilliance added depth to their discussions, and Vaibhav's playful energy brought a touch of excitement to their adventures.

As Vinay entered the 4th standard, his family received a special blessing—a baby girl. The news brought joy and happiness, but it also meant a shift in the family's dynamics and financial responsibilities. Vinay's parents had to be more cautious with their expenses to ensure they could meet the needs of their growing family. Despite being a young child, Vinay understood the situation and never burdened his father with unnecessary requests. He witnessed his parent's efforts to make ends meet and took it upon himself to contribute in any way he could. Vinay eagerly helped his mother with small household chores, alleviating some of her responsibilities and showing his support.

On Friday, as Vinay was attending school, his father, Mr. Sharma, unexpectedly arrived early to pick him up. With a smile on his face, Mr. Sharma shared the exciting news that Vinay's little sister had arrived. Overjoyed, Vinay couldn't contain his excitement, eager to meet his baby sister. Seeing Vinay's happiness, Vijay, his best friend, couldn't help but feel the desire to share in the joy of a new sibling as well. Gathering his courage, Vijay approached the teacher and requested leave for the day, explaining his wish to experience joy alongside Vinay. Acknowledging the bond between the two friends, the teacher granted Vijay's request, allowing him to accompany Vinay on this special day.

In contrast, Vaibhav, the mischievous child, also stood up and made a request for leave. However, his motives were different from Vinay and Vijay. Vaibhav simply wanted to escape the perceived monotony of the classroom. Understanding his true intentions, the teacher turned down Vaibhav's request, emphasizing the importance of attending school. However, Vaibhav was undeterred. He saw an opportunity and directly approached Mr. Sharma, requesting leave with a playful grin. Surprisingly, Mr. Sharma, recognizing the innocence of childhood, approved Vaibhav's request, understanding his desire to join his friends and share in the celebration. With the teacher's approval and Mr. Sharma's agreement, the four of them—Mr. Sharma, Vinay, Vijay, and Vaibhav—made their way to the hospital. Excitement filled the air as they embarked on this memorable journey together.

In that moment, the boundaries of friendship and family blended, as they embraced the joyous occasion of Vinay's sister's arrival. The bond between the three friends, strengthened by their shared experiences and understanding, allowed them to come together in celebration. In the following days, Vijay and Vaibhav became regular visitors to Vinay's house, eagerly seeking moments to spend time with the new baby. Vaibhav, realizing the benefits of their friendship, recognized that being in their company could provide him with advantages such as updated notes and favorable remarks from teachers. He relished the perks that came with their companionship.

One evening, as they sat together enjoying dinner at Vinay's house, Vaibhav enthusiastically broached the topic of an upcoming school trip. His eyes sparkled with excitement as he imagined the adventures and fun they could have together. Vaibhav's excitement continued to fill the room. He couldn't help but express his thoughts and dreams to his friends. "I can't wait for the school trip!" Vaibhav exclaimed, his voice brimming with anticipation. "Just imagine, guys, we'll be exploring new places, discovering fascinating sights, and creating memories that will last a lifetime. I can almost feel the rush of adrenaline as we embark on exciting adventures together." His imagination ran wild as he continued, "We'll be climbing mountains, splashing in clear blue waters, and maybe even encountering unique wildlife. I can already picture us laughing, cheering, and capturing every moment with our cameras. This trip will be the highlight of our school year!"

As the conversation progressed, Vinay's inner conflict became more evident, his gaze shifting to his parents, who were silently listening to the conversation. He understood the challenges they faced in managing their finances and didn't want to burden them further. At that moment, Vinay made the difficult decision to restrain himself, opting to quietly observe the discussion rather than express his own desire to join the trip. Vijay, loyal and understanding, respected Vinay's unspoken decision. He maintained his silence, offering his support through his quiet presence. He understood that true friendship meant being considerate of each other's circumstances and not pushing someone beyond their comfort zone. Vaibhav's excitement radiated through his words, as he envisioned the camaraderie and shared laughter that awaited them. He eagerly painted a vivid picture of the fun and thrills that lay ahead, completely absorbed in the anticipation of this new adventure. His friends listened, absorbing Vaibhav's contagious enthusiasm, even as they remained reserved in their own thoughts.

Within a week of anticipation, the teachers finally announced the much-awaited school trip that was scheduled to take place during the upcoming vacation. The destination was a picturesque hill station, promising three days of exploration and adventure. The cost per student was set at 1500/-. Vinay, determined not to burden his family with additional expenses, had already made up his mind not to be a part of the trip. Meanwhile, Vijay and Vaibhav, eager to embark on the exciting journey, promptly made their payment, eagerly securing their spots.

The following two months were dedicated to rigorous studies as the final exams approached. Vinay and Vijay, known for their academic excellence, continued to excel in their studies, consistently ranking at the top of their class. Their dedication and hard work were evident in their performance, and they earned the admiration and praise of their teachers. As the final day of the 4th standard approached, with just a week left before the highly anticipated trip, the teacher called Vinay aside for a special conversation. Vinay, a bit perplexed, approached the teacher, unsure of what awaited him. With a warm smile, the teacher spoke gently, "Vinay, I have wonderful news for you. In recognition of your exceptional academic achievements, I am pleased to inform you that you will be joining the school trip free of cost."

Vinay's eyes widened in disbelief, and a surge of joy coursed through his veins. The unexpected news overwhelmed him, and a wide smile stretched across his face. He could hardly contain his excitement as gratitude filled his heart. Overwhelmed with happiness, Vinay expressed his gratitude to the teacher, his voice filled with genuine appreciation. He couldn't believe his luck, feeling both honored and overjoyed to have the opportunity to be a part of the trip without placing any additional burden on his family. In that moment, Vinay's determination to be mindful of his family's financial situation had been rewarded with an unexpected blessing. The generosity and recognition from his teacher filled him with a sense of pride, validating his hard work and dedication. Vinay couldn't wait to share the news with his parents and friends, to see the smiles on their faces as they celebrated his achievement and the exciting adventure that awaited him. This unexpected turn of events added a new layer of excitement and anticipation to the trip, making it all the more meaningful.

One Week Later.

The morning sun peeked over the rolling hills as the students gathered, brimming with anticipation for their school trip. Excitement buzzed in the air as they boarded the buses, ready for an adventure-filled journey to the picturesque hill station.

As the buses ascended the winding mountain roads, the landscape transformed into a breathtaking panorama of lush greenery and cascading waterfalls. The students marveled at the majestic beauty unfolding before their eyes, their faces pressed against the windows, eager to take in every sight.

Upon reaching their destination, the students disembarked and were greeted by the refreshing mountain air. The trip organizers, with smiles on their faces, briefed the students on the itinerary and safety guidelines, ensuring that everyone was ready for the thrilling experiences ahead.

The first adventure awaited them at a nearby trekking trail. Led by experienced guides, the students hiked through dense forests, their laughter and chatter blending harmoniously with the sounds of nature. They maneuvered over rocky terrain, crossed gushing streams, and embraced the challenges with a zest for exploration.

Reaching a clearing at the summit, the students were rewarded with a breathtaking view of the valley below. A sense of accomplishment filled the air as they admired the panorama, their faces glowing with a mix of exhaustion and elation. The memory of conquering the trail would forever remain etched in their hearts.

Next on the itinerary was an adrenaline-pumping zip-lining experience. The students, adorned in safety gear, lined up with excited grins, ready to soar through the treetops.

As they launched off from the platforms, their screams of exhilaration echoed through the forest, merging with the sounds of nature. The wind rushed against their faces as they flew through the air, feeling a sense of freedom and awe at the breathtaking scenery below.

The adventure didn't end there. The students embarked on a river rafting expedition, navigating the frothy rapids with teamwork and excitement. Water splashed around them, and their laughter echoed across the river as they conquered each rapid with determination and camaraderie. The thrill of the adventure bonded them even further, fostering unforgettable memories and lifelong friendships.

As the sun began to set, the students gathered around a bonfire, sharing stories, laughter, and delicious snacks. They basked in the warmth of the fire, relishing in the sense of camaraderie and the spirit of adventure that had brought them together.

Underneath the starry night sky, the students engaged in a lively campfire sing-along, their voices harmonizing and filling the air with joy. As the embers glowed, they reflected on the incredible experiences of the day, feeling a deep sense of gratitude for the opportunity to explore, connect with nature, and forge unforgettable memories.

As the school trip drew to a close, the students returned to their buses, tired yet filled with a newfound sense of adventure and appreciation for the beauty of the natural world. The journey back home was filled with animated conversations, as they excitedly shared stories, laughed, and cherished the bonds that had grown stronger during their thrilling escapades.

A couple of years flew by, and now Vinay, Vijay, and Vaibhav found themselves in the final year of primary school. They stood at the precipice of teenagehood, a phase known for its complexities and challenges. Each of their fathers played an important role in their lives, providing guidance and support along the way. Vinay's father dedicated equal time to both his children, recognizing the importance of nurturing their individual growth. Mr. Sharma's love and care for Vinay were evident in the time he devoted to his son, ensuring he had the necessary resources and attention to flourish. Similarly, Mr. Patel made sure Vaibhav had all the resources he needed to explore his talents and interests. He encouraged his son to embrace his creativity and provided him with the tools to express himself freely. Vaibhav's father was determined to support his growth and help him navigate the complexities of adolescence. Meanwhile, Mr. Singh engaged in meaningful conversations with Vijay, staying updated on his experiences and accomplishments. He understood the significance of being involved in his son's life, providing him with a sense of security and a platform to express himself.

However, Vinay's parents found themselves facing a challenging situation. They realized that continuing Vinay's education at the same school might become financially burdensome. As they discussed the matter, unaware that Vijay was within earshot, they contemplated the possibility of transferring Vinay to a different school. Vijay, upon overhearing the conversation, felt his heartbreak. The thought of being separated from his dear friend, Vinay, weighed heavily on him. In a moment of despair, he approached Vinay's parents, pleading with them not to allow their friendship to be torn apart. Vijay couldn't fathom the idea of losing the companionship and support that Vinay had provided him throughout their shared journey. Mr. Sharma, Vinay's father, stood silent and helpless, understanding the pain his son and Vijay were experiencing. He recognized the profound bond between the two friends and the impact it had on their lives. However, the financial constraints and practical considerations presented a significant challenge that he wasn't sure how to overcome.

On that particular day, Vijay's usual bright smile was replaced with a cloud of sadness that enveloped his features. Sensing his friend's distress, Mr. Singh, Vijay's father, noticed the change in his son's demeanor and approached him with concern. He gently asked, "Vijay, my dear, what's troubling you today?" Vijay, with a heavy heart, poured out his worries to his father. He expressed his fear and concern about the possibility of Vinay being separated from their close-knit group of friends. Desperately seeking a solution, Vijay turned to his father, hoping for some guidance or a way to prevent this impending separation. Observing his son's genuine distress, Mr. Singh listened intently, his compassionate eyes reflecting understanding. Taking a moment to gather his thoughts, he spoke with a voice filled with empathy and wisdom.

"Vijay, my dear son, I understand how deeply this situation affects you. Life often presents us with circumstances that are beyond our control," Mr. Singh began, his tone gentle yet filled with a sense of realism. "Acceptance is a crucial aspect of life, my boy. It's important to understand that as we journey through life, we may face moments of detachment and separation from those we hold dear." Vijay's eyes filled with tears, yearning for a solution that would allow their friendship to remain intact. Mr. Singh, sensing his son's emotional turmoil, continued to offer his guidance and perspective.

"Remember, Vijay, the realities of life are such that we may not always have the power to influence certain outcomes. Sometimes, people may drift apart due to various reasons or circumstances. But true friendship is built on a foundation of love, trust, and shared experiences," Mr. Singh explained, his voice soothing. He continued,

"Although the prospect of separation is difficult to accept, it's important to understand that detachment is a part of everyone's journey. As we grow older, we encounter new experiences, meet new people, and venture onto different paths. It doesn't mean our friendships will diminish, but they may take on different forms and evolve in unexpected ways."

Listening intently to his father's words, Vijay gradually absorbed the wisdom imparted to him. While his heart still yearned for a resolution, he began to comprehend the inevitability of change and the importance of acceptance in life's journey. Mr. Singh lovingly placed a hand on Vijay's shoulder, offering comfort and reassurance. "My dear Vijay, no matter where life leads us, the memories we've created and the bond we share with Vinay will always remain within us. Our friendships have the strength to endure, even if circumstances change. Trust that your connection with Vinay will withstand the test of time."

Vijay, though still affected by the imminent separation, found solace in his father's words. He understood that while the future held uncertainty, the love and camaraderie he shared with his friends would endure the trials and tribulations of life. In that heartfelt moment, Vijay's spirits lifted slightly as he realized the importance of cherishing the moments they had together. He resolved to make the most of the time they had left, savoring each precious moment and holding onto the memories they had already created. Little did they know that life's journey would continue to unfold, presenting them with both challenges and opportunities. Vijay took solace in his father's wisdom, knowing that he had the strength and support to face whatever lay ahead, embracing the realities of life with acceptance and love.

As the reality of Vinay's impending departure from their school sank in, he mustered the courage to inform Vijay and

Vaibhav about his upcoming transfer. Vijay had already sensed this change brewing, so the news wasn't entirely surprising to him. However, for Vaibhav, the revelation came as a shock, momentarily leaving him speechless.

As the days unfolded, Vaibhav's reliance on Vinay became increasingly apparent, fueled by a deepening sense of worry. The upcoming departure of Vinay, a constant source of strength, left Vaibhav feeling exposed and unsettled. The thought of navigating upcoming challenges without Vinay's comforting presence began to chip away at Vaibhav's once unwavering confidence, introducing a tangible undercurrent of discomfort. Vaibhav, who was once self-assured and independent, now grappled with an unexpected vulnerability, starkly contrasting with the resilience he had always drawn from Vinay's steadfast support. The looming separation cast a shadow over Vaibhav's usual assurance, and the emptiness left by Vinay's impending absence disrupted the equilibrium of their friendship.

Vinay and Vijay, discerning the shift in Vaibhav's demeanor, decided to address the change directly. When confronted, Vaibhav opened up, admitting that Vaibhav felt really bad about himself. The thought of failing his exams made him sad all the time. Every day, the pressure of the exams got heavier, and he couldn't stop thinking about it. He always compared himself to his friends and worried that he might let his family down. The idea of failing scared him a lot.

One day, Vaibhav thought about cheating in the exams. He knew it was wrong, but he felt so desperate to avoid failing that he considered it. The more he thought about taking a shortcut, the more tempting it became.

He was stuck, not knowing what to do. He knew cheating was against what was right, but the fear of failing made him ignore that. It felt like he was standing at the edge of a big decision, not sure if he should step forward or not.

Vaibhav was scared of losing something, but he couldn't quite figure out what it was—maybe his dreams, feeling good about himself, or just the safety he used to have. The difference between what was right and wrong became blurry because of all the stress and doubt in his mind.

In response, Vinay, with a reassuring tone, spoke earnestly to his friend.

"Listen, Vaibhav," Vinay began, "there will be moments in life when external help might be scarce and situations may not unfold in our favor. It's during these times that we must trust in ourselves and possess a clear mind that can discern between right and wrong. You're inherently a good person, and that's why we chose you as our friend. Even if circumstances lead to a change in schools, it will never diminish the bond we share."

Vinay, understanding the importance of the upcoming exams for Vaibhav, suggested he concentrate on his studies. In a genuine attempt to seek assistance, Vaibhav turned to Vinay for help. However, an unfortunate twist occurred when a passing boy in the corridor misinterpreted their initial conversation. With a different narrative in mind, he swiftly complained to the teacher, inadvertently sparking a series of unintended consequences.

Considering the seriousness of the situation, she knew immediate action was necessary to address this breach of integrity. With a determined expression, the teacher, Miss Clarie, reached for the phone on her desk and dialed the number for Mr. Patel. After a brief conversation, Miss Clarie requested Mr. Patel's presence in her office. It was essential for him to hear firsthand what had unfolded. Moments later, Mr. Patel entered the room, his authoritative presence casting a shadow over the proceedings.

Miss Clarie relayed the entire incident to Mr. Patel, emphasizing the gravity of the situation. She urged him to take action against Vaibhav for his unacceptable behavior. However, to her surprise, Mr. Patel seemed skeptical, unable to believe the words of his trusted teacher. Vaibhav, who had been called to the office as well, seized the opportunity to defend himself. He vehemently denied any wrongdoing, painting himself as the victim in an elaborate lie. His words were convincing, causing doubt to creep into Mr. Patel's mind. The tension in the room escalated as a heated argument ensued. Mr. Patel's credibility was put into question, and the clash of perspectives intensified. Mr. Patel's unwavering faith in his son clouded his judgment, blinding him to the truth that lay before him. Struck by a mixture of disappointment and anger, Mr. Patel made a difficult decision and announced that his son Vaibhav would not continue pursuing one more year in the same school.

Takeaways:

★ Recognize academic achievements.

★ Encourage an inclusive environment where students feel a sense of belonging.

★ Promote positive peer relationships and support networks among students.

★ Implement support systems for students facing academic challenges.

★ Ensure disciplinary actions are fair and unbiased.

★ Encourage active participation of parents in their children's education.

Chapter 4

Paths of Transformation

"High school, a transformative journey where laughter and friendship echo through the halls, where choices shape not only careers but the essence of who we become."

High school is a time full of experiences that shape your future. It's an important point where your learning mixes with thinking about what job you want to do. This helps set the path you'll follow for your whole life. During these years, as you walk down the halls filled with laughter, friendships, and shared secrets, you also deal with changing feelings and figuring out who you are. Being a teenager means being curious and learning about yourself. This mixes with trying to do well in school and having big dreams. You might ask yourself, "What do I want to be when I grow up?" and "Who am I turning into?" High school is like a place where you test how strong you are and how well you can change. It's a time when you grow from being a kid to becoming an adult, bit by bit. In these years of growth, the good times and the tough times in high school don't just shape what job you'll do, but also what kind of person you'll be and how you'll handle the ever-changing world with more smarts.

Vinay's days were marked by a steady rhythm of responsibility. His role as a caregiver for his sister had become second nature, and he handled it with grace. Mornings were a whirlwind of getting his sister ready for school, ensuring she had her lunch, and then heading off to his own classes. Afternoons were a seamless transition from school to work, where he would assist his father with his tuition. Vinay's understanding of the world was growing rapidly, and with each passing day, he felt a deeper connection to his family's struggles. Despite the challenges, he found solace in his sister's smile and the sense of accomplishment that came from being a pillar of support.

Vijay, on the other hand, had found a new routine that provided him with some semblance of companionship. His visits to his father's office after school had transformed into a ritual. He helped with simple tasks, ran errands, and sometimes just sat beside his father as he worked. Through these moments, he gained insight into his father's dedication and work ethic. Vijay's loneliness gradually subsided, replaced by a growing sense of admiration for his father's commitment to providing for the family. However, a part of him still longed for the carefree days spent with his old friends.

Meanwhile, Vaibhav's path was taking a darker turn. The allure of immediate gratification was difficult to resist, and he often found himself making choices that he knew were wrong. He was drawn towards a group of peers who shared his mindset, and together, they embarked on adventures that pushed ethical boundaries. Skipping classes, engaging in minor raggings, and disregarding rules became their way of asserting control over their lives. Vaibhav's negative emotions seemed to find an outlet in this reckless behavior, temporarily filling the void he felt within.

Two years had slipped away, and now the trio stood on the precipice of their final year of high school. Time had wrought its changes, molding them in subtle yet significant ways. Through the ups and downs, one thread had remained unbroken – their Sunday hangouts. These weekly gatherings, once rooted in friendship, had transformed into a complex tapestry of emotions and motivations.

Vinay and Vijay, ever the steadfast companions, continued to meet for the genuine joy of friendship. The passage of time had only deepened their bond, and their conversations had evolved from the trivial to the profound. Each Sunday was a sanctuary, where they exchanged stories, and dreams, and laughed at old jokes as if time had stood still.

For Vaibhav, however, the Sunday gatherings bore a different significance. His attendance was tinged with a sense of obligation rather than enthusiasm. After the incident that led to a temporary separation within the trio, they had made a silent pact to avoid the topic altogether. Yet, that incident had left an indelible mark on Vaibhav's memory. Despite the passage of time, he could not shake off. He often found himself oscillating between thoughts of revenge and the practicality of maintaining connections that might serve his interests in the future.

The 10th standard had arrived, bringing with it a sense of urgency and expectation. Vinay, Vijay, and Vaibhav found themselves standing at the threshold of a crucial period in their lives. With each passing day, the pressure to make career decisions grew stronger, a chorus of voices urging them to shape their futures. The hallways were abuzz with talk of courses, colleges, and dreams waiting to be fulfilled. It was as if the world had suddenly magnified, demanding them to think about who they wanted to become.

However, the trio remained suspended in indecision, their dreams still blurry and undefined. Amidst the cacophony of advice, there was a constant, unwavering thought – the image of their fathers. Fathers who had worked hard, overcome challenges and stood as beacons of inspiration. For Vinay, it was the compassion with which his father dealt with people that stood out. For Vijay, his father's ability to lead with a blend of firmness and empathy was a guiding light. Vaibhav, on the other hand, marveled at his father's acumen in managing business and wielding authority.

As they walked this path of uncertainty, another wave hit them unexpectedly – the wave of love. It was during this year that they began to understand the complexity of their emotions. Crushes, infatuations, and the newfound awareness of romantic feelings added another layer of complexity to their already tangled thoughts. Just as they were grappling with the weight of career choices, they now found their hearts entangled in the web of teenage emotions.

With her elegance and striking features, Simran brought a fresh aura into their lives, instantly becoming a noticeable presence in their close-knit circle. Having recently relocated to the nearby society, she had joined Vinay's school in the final year – a year marked by uncertainties, yet an opportunity for new beginnings. As Simran grappled with the challenges of this transition, seeking solace in an unfamiliar environment, Vinay emerged as a helping hand, as recommended by their teachers.

Their interaction, initially driven by mutual need, effortlessly transformed into a genuine friendship. For Vinay, however, this connection transcended the boundaries of friendship. Simran wasn't just another friend; she was a person who ignited feelings he had never experienced before. His solitary moments were no longer solitary; Simran had become a part of his world, casting a warm glow on his thoughts.

Yet, even amidst this newfound happiness, there was an unexpected twist. One day, the rhythm of their meetings was disrupted. Vinay had always prioritized his friends, especially the Sunday hangouts that held a special place in his heart. However, when Simran requested his assistance in exploring the city, Vinay found himself in a dilemma. It was a sudden change of plans, one that surprised not only his friends but also himself. For the first time in two years, Vinay missed their regular gathering.

Curiosity and a hint of playfulness led Vijay to inquire about Vinay's sudden absence. Vinay revealed that he had been accompanying Simran on her city tour, leaving his friends both intrigued and amused by this newfound friendship. Vijay, always open and welcoming, saw an opportunity to expand their circle. He encouraged Vinay to introduce them to Simran, to embrace the chance of weaving their worlds together.

The moments shared with Simran were etching themselves into Vinay's heart as something truly special. He felt an urge to share this newfound connection, especially with Vijay, his confidant. In fact, he was beginning to wonder if this sensation he felt was indeed love.

Time with Simran seemed to move at a pace of its own, with a week vanishing like a fleeting moment. Their outings, filled with laughter and exploration, appeared to condense into mere minutes, leaving Vinay in awe of the depth of their conversations. He noticed that Simran's choices often mirrored his own, yet her mannerisms carried shades of Vijay. This amalgamation of familiarity made him feel at ease in her presence as if he had known her far longer than just a week.

Simran's open-mindedness resonated with Vinay, and their companionship had the power to transform mere days into cherished memories. One day, after their city tour, Simran embraced Vinay in a heartfelt hug, a gesture of gratitude for his guidance. For Simran, it was a simple act of thanking a friend, but for Vinay, that hug etched an indelible mark on his memory. It was as if the world stood still for that brief moment, allowing him to feel a warmth that lingered long after their embrace ended.

The day after their memorable outing, within the corridors of the school, Vinay found the courage to speak up. With a mix of anticipation and vulnerability, he shared with Simran that he had skipped the regular hangout with his friends to spend time with her. He explained how his friends were eager to meet her. Simran's eyes lit up with excitement as she absorbed this information, her curiosity piqued by the prospect of making new friends.

Intrigued by the idea, Simran leaned in and asked Vinay about his friends, especially about Vijay. Vinay's eyes sparkled as he painted a vivid picture of his friends, dwelling longer on Vijay's characteristics. He spoke of Vijay's openness, his infectious laughter, and his unique perspective on life. With each word, Vinay's enthusiasm was palpable, and Simran couldn't help but share in his excitement.

As Vinay talked about Vijay, Simran's interest grew, and her curiosity was now intertwined with a genuine eagerness to meet this person who held a significant place in Vinay's life. Vinay, sensing her interest, began to reveal stories about their adventures, their conversations, and the unbreakable bond they shared. Simran's anticipation for their upcoming meeting only intensified, and the prospect of making new friends in this unfamiliar place seemed more appealing than ever.

The day of the long-awaited meeting dawned, marked by an air of excitement and anticipation. As the trio gathered to meet Simran, her presence was a breath of fresh air. Dressed in a royal blue salwar kameez, she exuded an elegant aura that caught Vinay's breath with a single glance. His usual eloquence seemed to vanish, replaced by a stunned silence as he took in her appearance.

However, it was Simran who broke the ice with her enthusiasm. She confidently introduced herself and engaged in conversation with Vijay, her energy and openness instantly putting everyone at ease. While Vaibhav arrived a bit later, his entrance was nothing short of dramatic as his eyes widened upon seeing Simran. The day's dynamics shifted as they all settled in, eager to get to know one another.

Throughout the day, conversations flowed smoothly, akin to the rhythm of old friends catching up. Simran shared stories of her life, detailing her family's experiences of relocating due to her father's government job that led them to traverse four towns. Her admiration for Vinay and Vijay was evident, acknowledging the warmth and kindness they radiated.

As the interactions unfolded, Vaibhav, with his trademark charm, interjected with quirky questions that surprisingly added to the lighthearted atmosphere. His unexpected yet entertaining inquiries managed to steer the conversations into amusing territories. Through his jesting, Vaibhav brought an element of cheer to the gathering, showcasing the unique dynamics of their friendship.

In a culmination of shared laughter and exchanged stories, Simran, in a tone of genuine interest, inquired if she could join their hangout ritual from time to time. The response was unanimous and joyful, with everyone welcoming the idea.

Time flowed gently, and the bond between the four friends grew deeper with each passing day. Yet, amidst the laughter and shared moments, a quiet mystery lingered around Vinay. His feelings for Simran remained veiled, hidden behind a curtain of uncertainty. Vinay wasn't ready to rush to conclusions. His perspective on love was profound, a reflection of the enduring bond he had observed between his parents. He understood that love was a journey encompassing both sunny days and stormy nights.

Vinay's hesitation to reveal his emotions stemmed from a profound sense of responsibility. He didn't want to declare his feelings in the heat of the moment, only to later realize he had made a misjudgment. He valued Simran's emotions above all else and was committed to treading carefully. In his eyes, protecting her from any potential heartache was a priority, even if it meant he had to grapple with his own feelings.

Amidst these complex emotions, Vinay clung to a belief that resonated deeply with him – the notion that love was not something to be plucked like a flower. Instead, it was a delicate entity that required nurturing, just like watering a plant to let it bloom. He yearned to create a beautiful life for Simran, one where their love could flourish in the most genuine way possible.

Unbeknownst to him, Vinay was subconsciously painting a future with Simran in his mind. The dreams he wove, the care he took in building a foundation for their connection— all these actions were driven by a love that was profound and steadfast. As the days turned into weeks and weeks into months, Vinay was quietly nurturing the love in his heart, like a hidden garden waiting for the right moment to bloom.

Takeaways:

★ Reflect on personal growth; Consider your own high school experiences and how they contributed to your personal growth and future aspirations.

★ Evaluate friendships; Reflect on the dynamics of your friendships and how they've evolved over time, recognizing the impact of individual choices on group dynamics.

★ Embrace opportunities to form new connections, recognizing the potential for growth and enrichment in diverse relationships.

★ Envision the kind of future you want to build for yourself, drawing inspiration from the narrative's exploration of dreams, aspirations, and the pursuit of genuine connection.

Chapter 5

Whispers of the Heart

"Amidst the choices that shape our futures, the unexpected turns of friendship, and the complexities of love, the heart often surprises even the most cautious souls."

The board exams had come and gone, leaving in their wake a sense of accomplishment for Vinay and Vijay, as usual. These twin brothers had always been the pride of their families, consistently excelling in academics. However, this year held a pleasant surprise for everyone: their childhood friend, Vaibhav, had secured a first-class result. The joy was doubled when Simran, their close friend, joined in the celebrations with her own impressive achievement - a distinction.

The families couldn't have been happier. In a country where academic success was often seen as a ticket to a better future, their children had not disappointed them. The trio, Vinay, Vijay, and Vaibhav, sat together amidst the cheerful commotion, basking in their collective glory. However, the time had come for them to make important decisions about their future, and college was the next logical step.

The families had decided to take a progressive approach. They offered their children the freedom to choose their fields of study based on their interests. The young minds were excited at the prospect of making choices that would shape their careers. After some discussions, they settled on the field of commerce, believing it offered them a balanced mix of prospects and opportunities.

As they huddled around the dining table, laptops open, brochures scattered about, Simran entered the scene, her eyes shining with curiosity. She couldn't help but be drawn to the animated discussions about college choices.

"What are you guys up to?" she asked, her tone light and inquisitive.

Vaibhav, always the quickest to respond, looked up and grinned. "We're in the process of choosing our colleges. We've decided to go for commerce. You should join us!"

Vinay chimed in, "Yeah, it would be so much fun if we could all study together."

Simran appreciated the warmth of their invitation but politely declined. "Thank you both, but I've made up my mind. I'm leaning towards arts and literature."

Silence hung in the air for a moment, interrupted only by the soft hum of the ceiling fan. Simran's choice was unfamiliar territory for everyone. She had always been known as a bright student, but her passion for literature had remained a well-kept secret.

Vinay, who had always been the more outspoken of the two brothers, couldn't hide his disappointment entirely. "Are you sure, Simran? Commerce is a solid choice, and we could all be together."

Simran smiled at Vinay, her eyes twinkling with determination. "I appreciate the offer, but this is something I've always wanted to pursue. Literature and the arts have a special place in my heart."

As Simran's words settled in, it was Vijay's turn to speak. He leaned forward, his curiosity piqued. "Tell us more about your interest in arts and literature, Simran. We've known you for years, but this is something new."

Simran's face lit up as she spoke about her love for books, her fascination with storytelling, and the way literature had shaped her perspective on life. Her words were eloquent, and her passion was palpable. As she spoke, it became clear that her decision was not a sudden whim but the result of deep introspection and genuine enthusiasm.

Vinay, who had been initially disappointed, couldn't help but smile as he listened to her. Her passion was infectious, and he realized that Simran was making the right choice for herself.

As Vinay, Vaibhav, and Simran prepared to leave, Vijay kindly offered to drop Simran off at her home. She graciously accepted the offer, feeling grateful for the warmth of Vinay's family. As they walked together, Vijay initiated a conversation about Simran's reading journey, curious to learn more about her.

Simran smiled warmly and began to share her story. "Books have always been my companions," she said. "I was often the only child in a new neighborhood, and changing places frequently made it challenging for me to make friends during my childhood. So, I turned to books for solace and adventure. They opened up new worlds for me, and I've cherished them ever since."

Vijay nodded in understanding, appreciating the power of books to provide comfort during difficult times. He, too, had a deep connection to literature and was eager to share his own experiences. "I can relate," he said. "My father, Mr. Singh, has an incredible library at our home. He's collected books from various genres and eras over the years. It's a treasure trove of knowledge and stories."

Simran's eyes lit up with curiosity. "That sounds amazing," she replied. "I would love to visit your father's library someday. It must be a paradise for book lovers like us."

Vijay grinned, happy to have found a kindred spirit in Simran. "You're most welcome anytime," he said. "I'm sure my father would love to meet you and discuss books. Maybe we can plan a visit soon."

As they continued their walk, Simran and Vijay talked about their favorite books and authors, sharing stories and recommendations. Their connection deepened, and by the time they reached Simran's home, they felt like old friends. They exchanged contact information, promising to stay in touch and make plans for a visit to Vijay's home library.

Vijay was pleasantly surprised by how well he and Simran connected during their conversation. Her opinions on various topics resonated with him, and he couldn't help but feel a sense of kinship. It was rare for him to engage in such deep and meaningful discussions with someone other than his father, and he cherished this newfound connection.

Little did they know that this chance encounter and their shared love for books would lead to a beautiful friendship that would enrich both of their lives in the days to come.

As the college start date drew near, the bond between Vinay, Vijay, Simran, and Vaibhav had grown stronger. They had shared many memorable moments together, including a two-day trekking trip that Simran had enthusiastically organized. However, during this trip, Vaibhav couldn't help but notice that Simran seemed to be more involved with Vinay and Vijay. This observation triggered a brief moment of feeling left out and even a hint of jealousy in him.

Vaibhav was aware that he and Simran didn't share as many common interests as she did with Vinay and Vijay. He knew that their friendships had evolved differently, with Simran connecting on a deeper level. While Vaibhav enjoyed spending time with the group, he recognized that it was natural for people to have different connections and interests. Rather than dwelling on these negative emotions, Vaibhav chose to let them pass.

As time passed, the dynamics within their group became increasingly complex. Simran and Vijay's bond deepened through the exchange of books and discussions on various topics, including the concept of love. Vinay, who had noticed the growing connection between them, struggled with his own feelings. He cared deeply for Simran and was prepared to prioritize her happiness above all else. Love, he knew, had a way of making even the smallest thoughts lead to overthinking and sacrifices.

One evening, unable to contain his curiosity and concern, Vinay decided to broach the subject with Vijay. He asked, "Vijay, what are your feelings towards Simran?"

Vijay, caught off guard by the question, considered his response carefully. He knew that he had started to develop feelings for Simran, but he wasn't sure if he should label it as love. Their shared thoughts and tastes had drawn them closer, and he appreciated their compatibility. However, he also understood that not all close relationships needed to be romantic.

After a moment of contemplation, Vijay replied, "Vinay, I like Simran. I enjoy her company." Vinay, appreciating Vijay's honesty and sensitivity, nodded in agreement. He knew that their friendship was precious, and they would navigate these emotions with care. Little did Vijay and Vinay know that the path of their relationships was about to take an unexpected turn, as love has a way of surprising even the most cautious hearts.

Takeaways:

- ★ Consider the role of personal interests in shaping academic and career choices, and reflect on how these choices align with your passions and aspirations.

- ★ If facing decisions about your future, embrace the freedom to choose a path that aligns with your interests and aspirations, even if it deviates from conventional expectations.

- ★ In group dynamics, be aware of evolving relationships and feelings. Open and honest communication can help navigate complexities and maintain the integrity of friendships.

- ★ Prioritize the value of friendships and be open to understanding and respecting the feelings of others. Communication and empathy play crucial roles in preserving and nurturing relationships.

- ★ Acknowledge the unpredictable nature of emotions, especially in matters of the heart. Be open to unexpected turns in relationships and approach them with patience and understanding.

Chapter 6

Entangled Hearts

"We're all navigating our own unique maze of choices, and it's the sum of those choices that shapes our character."

On a typical weekend, Vijay and Simran found themselves at Vinay's house, engaging in their usual plans of relaxed conversations and tea. It was a ritual they cherished, a respite from the demands of their busy lives. Their gatherings at Vinay's place had become a sanctuary of sorts, where they could unwind, share stories, and delve into the topics that fascinated them.

However, this time, something seemed different. As they entered Vinay's cozy living room and settled into their familiar spots, Simran's demeanor caught their attention. She appeared a bit lost, her usually animated eyes clouded with thoughts.

Vijay, always perceptive when it came to Simran, couldn't help but notice her distant expression. He exchanged a quick glance with Vinay, silently acknowledging that something was on her mind. It was unusual for Simran to be so preoccupied during their weekend get-togethers.

Vinay offered Simran a warm cup of tea, hoping to break the silence that seemed to surround her. "Simran, is everything okay? You seem a bit preoccupied today."

Simran sighed, her gaze fixed on the steaming cup of tea in her hands. "Well, it's this assignment for my course," she began slowly. "I have to prepare a thesis on the psychology of humans and their duality, the gray area where they're neither entirely good nor entirely bad. It's been on my mind a lot, and I'm finding it quite challenging."

Vijay, who had always been drawn to profound topics and shared Simran's love for intellectual discussions, felt a spark of excitement. He leaned forward, his curiosity piqued. "You know, Simran, I've often pondered that same concept. In fact, it's something that's fascinated me for a long time."

Simran looked relieved to find a kindred spirit in Vijay. She turned to him, her eyes brightening with newfound enthusiasm. "You too? I thought I was the only one! It's like there's this inherent complexity in human nature that can't be neatly categorized as black or white."

Vinay, who had been quietly listening to their exchange, couldn't help but smile at the synchronicity of their thoughts. He settled back into his chair, content to let his friends delve into their discussion. After all, it was precisely these kinds of conversations that made their weekends so special.

Vijay continued, his words flowing with a sense of wonder, "It's as if we all carry within us this intricate blend of qualities, some admirable, and others not so much. But it's the choices we make that determine the shades of gray we inhabit."

Simran nodded thoughtfully, her gaze fixed on the wisps of steam rising from her tea. "Exactly, Vijay. It's in those moments of choice that our true colors shine through. Sometimes, it's the most unexpected people who surprise us with acts of great kindness, while those we think we know well may reveal darker aspects of themselves."

Vinay, now fully engaged in the conversation, leaned forward, his eyes bright with intellectual curiosity. "Isn't it fascinating how literature and psychology often explore this very theme? They provide us with a mirror to reflect upon the depths of human nature and the constant interplay between our light and dark sides."

As the discussion evolved, Vijay shared a personal story. "I remember reading a novel where the protagonist was this flawed character, caught in a moral dilemma. At first, I couldn't relate to their choices, but as the story unfolded, I found myself understanding their struggle. It was a powerful reminder that the gray areas of our own lives often need a closer look."

Simran added, "Yes, and sometimes, it's those very struggles and imperfections that make a character, or a person, relatable and ultimately endearing. We're all navigating our own unique maze of choices, and it's the sum of those choices that shapes our character."

Vinay chimed in, "It's not just about the choices we make but also the lessons we learn from them. The mistakes we've made and the moments of redemption all contribute to the evolving narrative of our lives."

The conversation between Vijay, Simran, and Vinay continued to deepen as they ventured further into the concept of the dual nature of human beings. Vijay, unable to contain his curiosity, leaned forward, his eyes filled with a hunger for understanding. "You know, Simran, it's not just about the individual. Society, too, has its own shades of gray when it comes to moral standards and values."

Simran's eyes met his, and she nodded thoughtfully, her mind racing with the implications of this broader perspective. "That's true, Vijay. Society's expectations often shape our decisions, and those expectations can be complex and contradictory. It's like we're constantly navigating a maze of conflicting norms, trying to find our way within this intricate web of collective morality."

Vinay, who had been silently absorbing their conversation, finally spoke up. His voice was measured, carrying the wisdom of someone who had pondered these questions deeply over time. "I've always believed that acknowledging our own duality and understanding it in others can lead to greater empathy and acceptance. It's a step towards a more compassionate world."

Simran's eyes brightened with realization, and a smile slowly spread across her face. "You're absolutely right, Vinay. This conversation has given me an idea for my thesis, one that could make it not just academically rigorous but also profoundly relevant to our lives. Instead of solely focusing on the individual's duality, I can explore how societal influences and cultural norms impact our perception of the gray areas in human nature."

Vijay and Vinay exchanged knowing glances, recognizing the brilliance of Simran's insight. Vinay applauded her idea, his enthusiasm matching Simran's. "That's a brilliant approach, Simran. By examining the interplay between the individual's inner complexities and the external pressures of society, you'll offer a holistic view of the human experience. It's not just about who we are as individuals; it's also about the world we live in."

As they continued to brainstorm and refine Simran's thesis idea, the room seemed to pulse with intellectual energy. Ideas flowed freely, and the boundaries between their individual thoughts blurred, creating a shared pool of knowledge and inspiration. Their discussion illuminated the intricate dance between the individual and society, shedding light on how the shades of gray in human nature were shaped, challenged, and molded by the world around them.

As Simran rushed off to her home, her excitement tangible in the air, Vijay and Vinay remained in Vinay's cozy living room, sipping their second round of tea. The room was bathed in a warm, golden glow from the soft lamplight, creating an atmosphere of intimacy and reflection. They both wore contented smiles, appreciating the presence of Simran and the profound discussions she always brought with her.

Vinay, who had been holding his feelings for Simran deep inside, felt a newfound sense of urgency to share his emotions with Vijay. He cleared his throat, choosing his words carefully. "You know, Vijay, Simran is such a thoughtful and sweet person that nobody can dislike her. She has this incredible ability to bring positivity into our lives, and I genuinely value her friendship."

Vijay, seemingly unaware of the hidden emotions behind Vinay's words, responded with his own revelation. His voice carried a mix of vulnerability and genuine affection as he spoke, "I think I have fallen for Simran. I don't know, Vinay, for me, all that matters is a connection and what I feel with her. The way we connect, as friends and on an intellectual level, it makes me want to spend the rest of my life with her."

Vijay's confession hung in the air like an unexpected storm, leaving Vinay momentarily stunned. He had not anticipated this revelation from his friend. The weight of his own unspoken feelings for Simran suddenly pressed heavily on his heart. It felt like a seismic shift in their friendship, and Vinay grappled with the uncertainty of how to respond.

Vinay's silence hung in the air like a heavy cloud as he listened to Vijay pouring his heart out about his feelings for Simran. He sat there, struggling to find words to express his own emotions, his heart aching with the weight of his unspoken love.

Once Vijay left for his own home, Vinay found himself alone in his apartment, engulfed by a deep sense of pain and turmoil. It was late in the evening, and the world outside had grown quiet, but Vinay had no appetite for dinner. He lay on his bed, tears welling up in his eyes but refusing to fall, mirroring the emotions that were trapped within him, just like his feelings for Simran.

In the darkness of his room, Vinay grappled with his inner turmoil. He couldn't quite decipher what hurt him more—the gnawing sense of insecurity or the knowledge that pursuing his love for Simran could potentially hurt his dear friend, Vijay. Vijay had always been a pillar of strength in Vinay's life, a friend he cherished deeply.

Vinay was caught in a relentless tug-of-war between his genuine affection for Simran, the blossoming love that had captivated his heart in recent months, and the unwavering loyalty he felt toward his friend Vijay. He knew that confessing his feelings to Simran could lead to a rift in their friendship, something he couldn't bear to imagine.

As the night wore on, Vinay's inner turmoil grew more profound. He had always believed in being honest with himself and others, but this was an unprecedented situation. Simran's rejection would undoubtedly bring sadness, but her acceptance also seemed like a double-edged sword, poised to cut deeply into Vijay's heart.

It was indeed a painful night for Vinay, a night filled with introspection and heartache. He lay there, wrestling with his emotions, wishing for a solution that would spare everyone involved from pain and heartbreak. The bonds of friendship, love, and loyalty had created a web of complexity that seemed impossible to untangle, leaving Vinay in a state of emotional turmoil that would not easily fade away.

Takeaways:

★ Read novels and works that delve into the complexities of human nature, drawing inspiration for personal growth and understanding.

★ Engage in discussions and research on societal norms and values, exploring the nuances of collective morality and its impact on individual choices.

★ Foster a culture of empathy and acceptance in personal relationships and within the broader community, recognizing and appreciating the diversity of human experiences.

★ Reflect on personal choices, acknowledging mistakes, and celebrating moments of growth and redemption as integral parts of the evolving narrative of life.

★ Initiate open and supportive conversations with friends, creating spaces for intellectual exchange and the sharing of thoughts and feelings.

★ Embrace personal growth and self-discovery, recognizing that the journey involves navigating shades of gray and evolving into a more authentic and compassionate self.

Chapter 7

Navigating Emotions

"Some connections are simply too precious to be defined by labels and expectations."

The next few months were hard for Vinay. Life had taken a twist he hadn't quite anticipated, and his emotions were running wild. It seemed like he was trapped in a never-ending rollercoaster ride, unable to control the ups and downs of his feelings.

Whenever he saw Vijay and Simran together, a sense of fear gripped him. It was an irrational fear of losing Simran, someone who had become an integral part of his life. Their bond had been strong, and he cherished the moments they had spent together. However, Vinay was also genuinely happy for his friend. Vijay had been his friend, and seeing him with someone as wonderful as Simran filled Vinay with a sense of contentment. There was no doubt in his mind that Vijay was the right guy for Simran.

Vinay had been trying his best to distance himself from Simran whenever Vijay was around, hoping to give them the space they needed to nurture their growing relationship. However, his efforts did not go unnoticed by the two people who mattered most to him - Simran and Vijay.

One day, as they found themselves in the same group again, Simran and Vijay decided to confront Vinay about his changing behavior. They cared about Vinay deeply, and they could see that something was bothering him.

Vinay, attempting to sound as casual as possible, explained, "I've known Simran since we were in the same school, and I just thought you two might want some time together. You have so many similarities and common topics to discuss, so I thought I'd give you space to vibe."

Simran looked at Vinay with a warm smile and replied, "Vinay, you were the first one to be my friend in this town, and our bond means the world to me. But I want you to understand something important. Just because we make new friends and connect with new people doesn't mean we lose the connections we already have. You've been an essential part of my life for so long, and that's not going to change."

Vijay, realizing the reason behind Vinay's changed behavior, chimed in, "Vinay, I also cherish the friendship we share. I may have more topics to discuss with Simran, but that doesn't overshadow the bond we have with you. We're not here to replace anyone; we're here to create new connections and share our lives with the people we care about."

Hearing these heartfelt words from Simran and Vijay, Vinay felt a wave of emotions wash over him. He realized that his fear of losing his friendship with Simran had been unfounded. Their bond was strong and enduring, and he didn't need to distance himself to make room for someone new. It was a moment of reassurance and clarity for all three friends.

As the evening sun cast a warm glow on the group, Vaibhav suddenly appeared on the scene, joining Simran and Vijay. Vinay, who had been feeling emotional and overwhelmed by the situation, saw an opportunity to have some time to himself. He turned to Vaibhav and, trying to sound nonchalant, said, "Hey Vaibhav, I just realized I have something urgent to attend to at home. Could you drop me off?"

Vaibhav agreed without hesitation, although he had just come. Vinay and Vaibhav left the group, leaving Simran and Vijay alone.

Simran, genuinely concerned about Vinay, turned to Vijay and asked, "Vijay, do you know if there's something bothering Vinay that he hasn't shared with me? Is there something I don't know?"

Vijay recognized Simran's worry and decided it was time to be honest with her. He began to explain the situation, recounting his conversation with Vinay where he had confessed his feelings for Simran, believing she would understand.

Listening carefully, Simran absorbed Vijay's words. When he finished, she smiled warmly and replied, "Vijay, I truly appreciate your honesty, and I want you to know how special you are to me. The bond we share is unlike any other, and I treasure it deeply. In fact, I can say that I like you the most. The connection I have with you, I haven't found with anyone else."

Vijay nodded in agreement, understanding the depth of their friendship. Simran continued, searching for the most polite way to express her thoughts. "But….." As Simran was saying, Vijay, understanding the situation, completed her words, stating, "But not every relationship needs to take the form of a couple friendship." Vijay began, his words filled with wisdom. "We can be friends and still have the same beautiful bond. I can still like you but without any expectation of getting myself chosen. And we can still love people without making it complicated."

Relieved and touched by Vijay's understanding and maturity, Simran hugged him tightly. She couldn't have asked for a better friend and was grateful that their bond was strong enough to withstand such situations.

Their friendship remained unshaken, proving that some connections were simply too precious to be defined by labels and expectations. They had a beautiful bond that transcended the boundaries of love, and it was something they both cherished dearly.

As a few months passed, life settled back into its familiar rhythm for Vinay and his friends. The same old days returned, where they would spend weekends together, enjoying each other's company. Vinay, who had needed some time to collect his thoughts and emotions, was back to his usual self. He felt supported by his friends, especially Vaibhav, who would often keep him company whenever he noticed Vinay was alone. Meanwhile, Vijay and Simran's bond had become even stronger with a newfound clarity in their boundaries.

However, Simran couldn't help but miss her days spent with Vinay. She cherished the memories of their time together, and those moments remained close to her heart. Often, she would visit Vinay's home unexpectedly, seeking the comfort and companionship of her first friend. Those impromptu visits with Vinay became her happiest moments, and the bond between them continued to grow stronger.

Vinay, although appreciative of Simran's visits, began to feel that he should provide more space for Vijay to be with her. He understood that the moments they shared now were essential for building their romantic relationship, and he didn't want to stand in the way of their happiness. It was a testament to Vinay's selflessness and his desire to see his friends' relationships thrive.

In the later 20's, Life in a Metro was doing well in theatres. Simran wanted to see that movie with her friends and was excited for the weekend. On the day of the planned movie outing, everything seemed set until Vaibhav had to attend to an unexpected guest at his home, forcing him to cancel his plans at the last minute. This sudden change left the trio of Vinay, Vijay, and Simran with a decision to make about whether to go to the movie without Vaibhav.

Vinay, considering the opportunity for Vijay and Simran to spend time together, thought of stepping back from the plan. As he began to excuse himself, he noticed a glint of moisture in Simran's eyes. Her reaction caught him by surprise, and before he could fully grasp the situation, Simran hurriedly left for her home, leaving Vinay and Vijay alone.

In that moment, Vinay and Vijay found themselves in an open and honest conversation. Vijay confessed that the romantic relationship between him and Simran was not what it seemed. They shared a deep and cherished friendship but didn't see any potential for a romantic relationship. The words were unexpected for Vinay, and he realized the consequences of his actions. Vinay had genuinely wanted to give Vijay and Simran a chance to spend time together, believing that it would strengthen their bond. However, his actions had inadvertently hurt Simran.

Vinay, realizing the depth of hurt he had inadvertently caused Simran, rushed to her house to console her. However, Simran's constant feelings of being ignored and disappointed were evident. Despite his sincere attempts to make amends, he found himself unable to console her, and a heavy silence hung in the air.

Finally, Simran broke the silence. She spoke candidly, saying, "I understand the reason behind your change in behavior, but it doesn't justify it in my eyes. We're friends, Vinay, and honesty is what I expect from you. Just as I respect your bonds with Vijay and Vaibhav, I expect the same respect for my relationships."

Vinay hesitated for a moment but eventually began, "It wasn't easy for me, but..." Simran interrupted, asking, "But what?"

"It's just that I wanted to give you and Vijay some space, and..." Vinay tried to explain, but Simran's response cut through his words: "We are just friends, Vinay."

"Yes," Vinay replied, "but Vijay is a nice boy, and he likes you, Simran."

Simran's next words questioned the entire perspective. "Vijay is a nice boy; that's undeniable. But is it sufficient for one person to enter into a relationship? Just because Vijay is a nice person, does my consent hold no importance? What if I am in love with someone else? If you had known, would you have still behaved the same way?"

Vinay was left speechless, unsure of how to respond. With a trembling voice, he managed to ask, "Are you in love with..." But before he could finish his question, Simran responded with a simple "yes."

"I'm sorry for not understanding or having an open conversation with you, Simran. I'm sorry, and I'll take my leave," Vinay admitted.

However, Simran grabbed his hand and asked, "Don't you want to know who it is?"

Vinay, overwhelmed by the situation, replied, "No, not today."

Simran insisted, "Why not? Why is it painful for you to hear the answer? Do you have anything to confess?"

Vinay found himself at a loss for words, unable to respond to Simran's direct questioning. The room was filled with the weight of unspoken feelings, leaving both of them in a state of emotional turmoil.

Simran's bold confession hung in the air, and Vinay was left speechless. It was something he had never anticipated hearing, especially in the midst of the turmoil that had unfolded. "But... Vijay," Vinay almost whispered.

"Vijay will understand it, and I want to know, do you understand my feelings?" Simran stood there, anticipation in her eyes, her own emotions more expressive than she had ever imagined. Vinay began, "The day I saw you was the day I started liking you, and slowly, unknowingly, I fell for you. But Vijay being in love.." His sentence remained incomplete, mirroring his inner conflict.

Simran responded with a gentle smile and said, "Go home, Vinay. We're all going to the movies together tomorrow—you, me, Vijay, and Vaibhav."

As Vinay left her house, he was filled with mixed emotions. He was undoubtedly happy to know that Simran liked him, but the thought of how it might affect Vijay's happiness weighed on him. Vinay's personality was gradually taking shape as he navigated the complexities of emotions, relationships, and his ideals.

Idealistic individuals often possess characteristics such as a strong sense of fairness, a deep commitment to their principles, and a desire to do what's morally right. They believe in the best in people and situations, striving to create a world that aligns with their values. Vinay's idealistic nature played a significant role in the moral and ethical dilemmas he faced, leading him to contemplate not just his own feelings but also the happiness and well-being of those around him, especially his close friends.

Takeaways:

★ Recognize and respect the boundaries in friendships and relationships, ensuring that individual connections are valued and maintained.

★ Encourage self-awareness and understanding of one's own feelings, as well as empathy for the feelings of others.

★ Provide support and understanding for friends navigating complex emotions, acknowledging that relationships can be nuanced and multifaceted.

★ Navigate the intersection of idealism and reality, recognizing that while ideals are important, relationships require flexibility and understanding of the complexities involved.

★ Embrace personal growth and self-discovery, understanding that navigating emotions and relationships contributes to individual development and maturity.

Chapter 8

Crossroads of Destiny

"The right choice is the one that aligns with your aspirations and values."

In the wake of Vinay and Simran finding happiness in their shared journey, life took on a wonderfully smooth rhythm for the couple. When the news of their budding relationship unfolded within the close-knit circle of Vijay and Vaibhav, the atmosphere brimmed with genuine joy. Vinay, mindful of Vijay's reaction, was pleasantly surprised to discover that Vijay's response exceeded his expectations. Vijay, showcasing an impressive level of maturity, not only retained their friendship but also warmly embraced the news, underscoring the depth of his understanding nature.

Vaibhav, a spectator to this newfound chapter in his friends' lives, experienced a unique emotion as he witnessed them falling in love. For the first time, he felt a subtle tug of desire to embark on his own romantic journey, yet he opted to let fate unfold its course naturally. The dynamics of their friendship, a cornerstone of their shared experiences, remained steadfast.

As they all continued their educational journey, years seemed to slip away like sand through their fingers. Before they knew it, they found themselves in the last year of their respective graduations. The final year brought with it a mix of emotions—fears of the unknown mingled with the palpable excitement of reaching a significant milestone.

For Vinay, Simran, Vijay, and Vaibhav, the prospect of graduation marked the culmination of an era filled with late-night study sessions, shared laughter, and the forging of lasting friendships. As they attended their last classes and prepared for final exams, the weight of the impending transition to the next chapter of their lives hung in the air.

The uncertainty of what lay beyond graduation stirred a certain level of fear. What career paths would they choose? Where would life take them? These questions loomed large, casting a shadow of apprehension over the otherwise celebratory atmosphere. The familiarity of the routine they had grown accustomed to was about to give way to the uncharted territory of adulthood.

Yet, amidst the fears of the unknown, there was an undeniable excitement. Graduation represented not only an academic achievement but also the doorway to new opportunities and experiences. The joy of completing a significant chapter in their lives mingled with the anticipation of what awaited them in the world beyond academia.

One night, as the campus selections loomed just a week away, a palpable tension hung in the air, particularly for Vaibhav. While Vinay and Vijay were driven by their ambitions to secure positions through the campus selections, Vaibhav, coming from a family rooted in business, found himself caught in a web of uncertainty.

Sensing his son's inner turmoil, Vaibhav's father decided it was time for a heart-to-heart conversation. Seated in the quiet of their home, the father looked at his son and said, "Vaibhav, I've noticed a certain confusion in your eyes. The campus selections are just around the corner, and I can see that you're grappling with a decision. Let's talk about it."

Vaibhav, appreciating the opportunity to share his thoughts, hesitated for a moment before expressing, "Dad,

I've been thinking a lot about whether to join the business or work for a company. It's not an easy choice for me. I see the success of our family business, but at the same time, I feel the pull to gain experience elsewhere. I'm not sure what's the right path for me."

His father, understanding the weight of the decision, spoke with a reassuring tone, "Vaibhav, life is a journey, and each path you choose offers its own set of experiences. It's completely normal to feel torn between the known and the unknown. What's important is that you follow your heart and gather experiences that will shape your understanding of the world. It's okay not to have all the answers right now."

Vaibhav, comforted by his father's wisdom, asked, "But Dad, how do I decide? I want to make the right choice."

His father smiled and replied, "The right choice, my son, is the one that aligns with your aspirations and values. Sometimes, you have to step out of your comfort zone to truly discover your strengths and passions. Consider working for a couple of years. It will give you a taste of the corporate world, and you might find clarity in the process."

Vaibhav, taking in his father's words, felt a sense of reassurance. The conversation ended with a decision forming in Vaibhav's mind. He nodded. "You're right, Dad. I'll work for a couple of years, gain some experience, and then decide. It's time for me to explore the unknown."

As father and son shared a moment of understanding, a new chapter in Vaibhav's life began to unfold—one that held the promise of valuable experiences and self-discovery.

On the other hand, as the campus selections drew near, Vinay found himself in a candid conversation with both his mother and father. There was a sense of responsibility that weighed on Vinay's shoulders, a desire to contribute to his family's well-being.

Shades of Life

Seated in the familiar surroundings of their home, Vinay took a deep breath before broaching the subject. "Mom, Dad, I've been thinking a lot about the future, especially with the campus selections approaching. I feel a responsibility towards the family, and I want to make sure I can contribute in the best way possible."

His mother, with a comforting smile, responded, "Vinay, we appreciate your sense of responsibility, but we also want you to prioritize your dreams and aspirations. Your well-being is just as important to us. What's on your mind?"

Vinay, opening up about his concerns, confessed, "I want to secure a good job to ensure stability for us. But I also feel the pressure to make the right financial choices. It's a bit overwhelming."

His father, understanding the weight of Vinay's words, spoke with a reassuring tone, "Vinay, we believe in you. You've always been hardworking and responsible. It's natural to feel the weight of these decisions, but don't forget to trust yourself. Money is one aspect, but it's not the only measure of success or happiness. Your well-being, satisfaction, and the alignment of your job with your values matter just as much."

His mother added, "We're here to support you, Vinay. Your happiness and fulfillment are important to us. Don't choose something solely for the sake of financial security. Follow your heart and pursue a path that resonates with who you are."

Vinay, feeling the warmth of his family's support, nodded. "Thank you, Mom and Dad. I needed to hear that. I want to choose a position or a job that not only provides security but also aligns with who I am."

His father, offering a final piece of advice, said, "Vinay, sometimes the value of a job goes beyond the paycheck. Consider factors like job satisfaction, personal growth, and how well they align with your personality. Choose a path that brings you fulfillment, and success will follow."

Vinay left the conversation with newfound clarity and determination. The support and guidance from his family eased the burden on his shoulders, allowing him to approach the upcoming decisions with a balanced perspective. As the campus selections loomed closer, Vinay felt a renewed sense of confidence, ready to embark on a path that blended financial security with personal fulfillment.

Unlike Vinay and Vaibhav, as the crucial time for campus selections approached, Vijay remained remarkably calm and composed, displaying a demeanor that caught the attention of his father, Mr. Singh. Sensing an opportunity for a meaningful conversation, Mr. Singh decided to share some insights with his son, acknowledging the reflective qualities he saw in Vijay.

One evening, as they sat together, Mr. Singh began, "Vijay, I've observed your calm and composed approach towards the upcoming campus selections. It reminds me of my younger self, and I thought it was time we had a conversation about what lies ahead."

Vijay, with a respectful nod, welcomed the discussion. Mr. Singh continued, "I've always admired your ability to face challenges with a clear mind. It's a valuable trait, and I can see that you've learned a lot from it."

Vijay humbly replied, "Thank you, Dad. I've had a great teacher."

Mr. Singh smiled. "It warms my heart to hear that. But, Vijay, I want you to know that while having ideals is commendable, it's equally important to forge your own path and make your own identity. I've always believed in leading by example, but I also encourage you to carve out your unique journey."

Shades of Life

Vijay, appreciating the wisdom in his father's words, shared, "I understand, Dad. I've learned a lot from you, and I aim to build my own identity while staying true to the values you've instilled in me."

At that moment, Vijay's mother, having overheard the conversation, joined in, saying, "Vijay, your father has always been an exemplary figure, but remember, your journey is yours alone. You have your own strengths, and I believe you'll make choices that reflect your character."

Vijay, feeling the support from both his parents, smiled and said, "Thank you, Mom. Thank you, Dad. I feel ready for whatever lies ahead."

Mr. Singh, proud of the composed and mature individual his son had become, concluded, "Vijay, go out there and do your best. Life is a journey, and a beautiful one awaits you. Embrace the challenges, learn from them, and remember, you have the power to shape your destiny."

As the conversation concluded, the Singh family shared a moment of unity and encouragement, with the assurance that Vijay was well-prepared for the journey that awaited him.

A week later, the much-anticipated campus selections unfolded, and the trio—Vinay, Vijay, and Vaibhav—each embarked on distinct paths in the professional world.

Vinay's exceptional punctuality and commendable track record led him to secure a position as a performance intern at a digital marketing firm. His skills in maintaining precision and dedication had not gone unnoticed, earning him a spot in a company that valued these qualities.

Vijay, with a vision to gain diverse exposure, opted for an internship at a content curation firm. This firm boasted an extensive client base, promising Vijay the chance to delve into various aspects of content creation and curation. It was a strategic move to broaden his horizons and gather experience from different corners of the industry.

In a deviation from the conventional path, Vaibhav decided to forgo the allure of multinational companies during campus selections. Driven by a fervor for gaining hands-on experience, he chose to work with a startup that specialized in fashion textiles, specifically in the production department. For Vaibhav, the startup scene offered a unique opportunity to understand the intricacies of the industry from the ground up.

Later that evening, the gang—Vinay, Vaibhav, Vijay, and Simran—gathered to share the exciting news. Laughter and joy filled the room as each of them recounted their success in the campus selections. Simran joined the celebration with her own achievement, securing an internship at a prestigious hospital. It was indeed a time for celebration, and they couldn't be happier for each other. The air buzzed with positivity, and their families, sharing in the joy, were equally overjoyed at the accomplishments of these young minds.

Takeaways:

★ Encourage individuals to explore the unknown, step out of their comfort zones, and gather diverse experiences that contribute to personal and professional growth.

★ Acknowledge the importance of financial stability while making career choices, but emphasize that it's not the sole measure of success or happiness.

★ Highlight the importance of maintaining composure and a clear mind during challenging times, emphasizing the power of resilience and a positive mindset.

★ Embrace the uncertainties and changes that come with transitions, emphasizing that they are part of life's journey and opportunities for growth.

★ Encourage seeking guidance from experienced individuals, such as parents, and valuing their wisdom while recognizing the importance of personal decision-making.

★ Inspire individuals to set aspirational goals, pursue their dreams, and be open to diverse opportunities that contribute to a fulfilling and meaningful life journey.

Chapter 9

Professionally Unraveled

"It's not a matter of right or wrong. It's about understanding what you want and recognizing the lessons life is weaving into your journey."

Vinay's work demanded nothing short of his complete attention, and he thrived in that demanding environment. His role seemed tailor-made for him, with his sharp eyes and analytical brain leaving no detail unnoticed. His approach to work was nothing short of idealistic, always striving to find the most effective ways to deliver results.

In the realm of performance, Vinay emerged as the cream of the crop. His actions were guided not just by the pursuit of profit for the company but also by a deep commitment to customer satisfaction. He believed in measures that not only brought tangible results but also ensured that customers were content with the outcomes.

His impact was felt soon after he joined. The company, under his watch, managed to not only attract but also retain customers. Vinay's knack for achieving desired results while keeping customer satisfaction at the forefront marked him as a standout performer. His dedication and exemplary work ethic were recognized when, in the span of 3 years of joining, he not only cleared probation but also found himself leading a team of performance interns.

Vinay not only led his team with great spirit but also contributed to making the company one of the most popular firms in Mumbai. The city's bustling nature, always attracting crowds and businesses, found Vinay an asset that stood out. His dedication to work with a strong ethical foundation proved to be the driving force behind his success.

As Vinay completed five years at the firm, the company decided to honor him with a small celebration. However, before he could join the festivities, his boss invited him into the cabin for a surprising conversation. "Vinay, first of all, congratulations. You've brought us considerable fame," the boss praised.

"Thank you, sir. It's my duty," Vinay replied humbly.

The boss continued, "In these five years, I've noticed something special in you, Vinay. You're not just a top performer; you're also an adept planner. You understand people and devise strategies that align with our goals. I firmly believe you should be given the chance to explore strategic planning. I want you to lead the department as the head, where you'll have the authority to decide on campaigns entirely."

Vinay was taken aback; he had never expected such a high position. In terms of hierarchy, he was promoted to the second-highest position in the company, just below the CEO. This promotion also came with a tremendous hike. The celebration that followed was filled with laughter and joy. When Vinay shared the news with his family and friends, everyone felt an overwhelming sense of pride for his remarkable achievement. The unexpected promotion was not just a recognition of his past success but also a testament to the trust and confidence the company had in his abilities.

Vijay's work led him on a fascinating journey through various industries, offering him exposure that expanded his horizons. His role gave him the opportunity to delve deeply into the world of content, a realm he cherished as an avid reader. His ability to think from multiple perspectives became a significant asset, propelling him to excel in his job.

Vijay's suggestions in the workplace were more than just ideas; they were gems that were often appreciated by his colleagues and superiors alike. He found immense satisfaction in being surrounded by intellectual individuals who shared his passion for creative and strategic thinking.

What truly set Vijay apart was his unwavering team spirit. In every project, he made sure his team received equal credit for their collective efforts. This selfless approach didn't go unnoticed by his superiors, who painted him as someone with leadership qualities. Vijay embodied the essence of a true team player, understanding that success is best achieved together. His dedication to lifting others up demonstrated not only his professional prowess but also his character, making him stand out as a natural leader in the workplace.

Vijay found himself frequently chosen to lead his team, a testament to the respect and trust his colleagues placed in him. One particular instance showcased Vijay's exceptional skills when faced with a conflict of creative differences between the company and a client. His diplomatic and calm approach not only resolved the issue but also saved the company's reputation.

As time passed, Vijay's superiors began to recognize that he wasn't just a leader with diplomatic skills; he embodied ethics and displayed a smart attitude necessary for higher levels of professionalism. Vijay consistently found himself involved in negotiations and client meetings, where his presentations and communication were not just on point but also instrumental in securing deals.

Unlike Vinay, whose performance often garnered immediate public reactions, Vijay's achievements were not as overt but certainly not unnoticed. It became evident that Vijay was quietly preparing for something bigger, with his strategic and ethical leadership setting the stage for future professional milestones. His journey was marked by a steady ascent, each accomplishment laying the foundation for what seemed like a promising future in the professional realm.

Vaibhav's journey in the professional realm turned out to be a rollercoaster of ups and downs. Stepping into the firm, he quickly realized that the business dynamics here were vastly different from the textile production his family was engaged in. While his family dealt with the consistent production of textiles, the industry he was currently navigating was marked by constant shifts in trends.

It wasn't just about production for Vaibhav; it was about the relentless pressure to meet demands and effectively sell the produced slots in a market that thrived on change. In response to these challenges, Vaibhav voluntarily stepped into leadership roles. He found himself wearing multiple hats, from overseeing production to delving into trend research. At times, he even had to take on the role of a salesperson, acting as an agent for the products.

Certainly, these responsibilities didn't all unfold at once, but each day brought with it new challenges for Vaibhav. Vaibhav's journey came with its fair share of sacrifices—late nights at work, postponed hangouts with friends—but he accepted these changes as part of the entrepreneurial grind. However, there were moments that tested his resolve, like when a potential client opted for another firm, leaving him heartbroken. In those low moments, he turned to his friends Vinay and Vijay, seeking solace.

In the dimly lit room, the weight of Vaibhav's uncertainties hung heavy in the air. As he questioned the path he had chosen, the flickering candlelight mirrored the flickers of doubt in his eyes. "Did I make the wrong decision?" he mused aloud, his voice echoing his internal struggle. Both Vinay and Vijay, perceptive to their friend's turmoil, leaned in, ready to offer the solace he sought.

Vinay, leaning back thoughtfully, began to dissect Vaibhav's concerns. "Vaibhav, my friend, it's not a matter of right or wrong. It's about understanding what you want and recognizing the lessons life is weaving into your journey. These struggles you're facing now, without significant monetary losses, are the building blocks for the challenges that lie ahead. You're not just in business; you're in a fiercely competitive industry."

Listening intently, Vijay, known for his calm demeanor, interjected with a touch of wisdom. "Vaibhav, life is like a chess game. Your moves now are shaping the board for the future. Embrace these challenges, learn from them, and you'll emerge stronger. Remember, success often comes after overcoming failures. It's all part of the game."

Vaibhav, grappling with the weight of his decisions, absorbed their insights. "But what if I can't handle the pressure and the constant uncertainty?" he questioned, seeking reassurance. Vinay, flashing a reassuring smile, replied, "Vaibhav, pressure and uncertainty are constants in any venture. It's about how you navigate through them. You have the resilience within you; tap into it. And remember, we're here for you, not just as friends but as partners in this journey."

The room, once filled with doubt, now echoed with the warmth of shared wisdom. These conversations, woven with genuine concern and advice, became the threads that strengthened the fabric of their friendship. As they continued to discuss life beyond the professional corner, the flickers of doubt gradually transformed into sparks of renewed determination for Vaibhav.

Vijay, observing Vinay's insightful guidance, chimed in, suggesting that Vaibhav should resume regular meetups with them. Feeling reassured by Vinay's advice, Vaibhav agreed to Vijay's suggestion. Vijay's recommendation wasn't just based on their friendship bond; as a visionary leader, he had observed something that others might have overlooked.

Takeaways:

★ Encourage an idealistic approach to work, always striving for effectiveness.

★ Adopt customer-centric approaches in attracting and retaining clients.

★ Promote dedication and exemplary work ethic as pathways to career recognition.

★ Inspire selfless leadership by giving credit to the team for collective efforts.

★ Emphasize the necessity of resilience in the face of uncertainties.

★ Encourage individuals to view challenges as opportunities for skill development.

★ Encourage individuals to have a vision for their professional journeys and take steps to realize it.

Chapter 10

Celebration of Bonds

> *"Let's not confine ourselves to societal norms that dictate these comparisons. We are individuals, and a marriage should never be built on such benchmarks."*

In the span of almost four years, Simran had traversed a remarkable journey, culminating in the successful establishment of her own clinic after completing her internship. Despite the prevailing norms that downplayed the significance of mental health, Simran boldly chose clinical psychology as her field of expertise in Mumbai. In a time where mental well-being wasn't given the attention it deserved, she embarked on a mission to normalize and prioritize it in society.

Simran's approach to clinical psychology went beyond the traditional confines of her profession. Recognizing that many individuals sought not only clinical help but also guidance for the unanswered dilemmas in their lives, she expanded her role. Through meticulous research and genuine care, she dedicated time to consulting people, particularly students, on their career and life decisions. Simran emerged as more than just a psychologist; she became a trusted advisor, understanding the intricate link between unanswered questions and the potential for a disturbed state of mind.

With an aura that exuded confidence and a demeanor that could confront anyone, Simran was not just breaking barriers in her profession but also actively contributing to reshaping societal perspectives on mental health.

Simran's clinic achieved unprecedented popularity when she took on the case of a Bollywood actress grappling with mental illness amid a series of constant failures. Through a series of consultations, Simran provided not just clinical support but also valuable life advice. Recognizing the challenges the actress faced in the film industry, Simran suggested exploring opportunities in serials if the film avenue wasn't proving fruitful.

Taking Simran's advice to heart, the actress transitioned to the world of television, marking a significant turning point in her career. The serial garnered immense popularity, and the actress, once on the brink of despair, made a triumphant comeback. In a poignant moment at an awards ceremony, the actress, holding her trophy, called Simran onto the stage to express her heartfelt gratitude.

This turning point not only showcased Simran's expertise in mental health but also highlighted her ability to offer practical and impactful advice beyond the realm of clinical psychology. The actress's public acknowledgment of Simran's role in her journey catapulted Simran into the spotlight, making her an unstoppable force in her field. As news of this success story spread, Simran's clinic became a sought-after destination for those seeking not just professional help but also life-altering guidance.

Amidst Simran's hectic schedules, she managed to strike a delicate balance between her personal and professional life. As the sands of time continued to slip away, her parents gently broached the topic of her marriage, expressing their desire for her to find a life partner. To their delight, Simran revealed that she and Vinay had been in love for years and that she wished to marry him.

Her parents were acquainted with Vinay, having known him since their relocation to Mumbai. They were well aware of his commendable qualities, and he, too, was excelling in his career. However, out of concern for their daughter's future, they cautiously suggested Simran reconsider her decision. They proposed the idea of exploring potential life partners within the same industry, thinking it might offer more stability and compatibility. In response, Simran, with a gentle but firm demeanor, expressed her resistance to conventional norms.

"Mom, Dad, it's not a prerequisite for a man to always outearn or be ahead of his wife. Vinay and I are both doing well in our respective fields and even if we weren't, we could always support each other. Let's not confine ourselves to societal norms that dictate these comparisons. We are individuals, and a marriage should never be built on such benchmarks," Simran asserted, defending her choice with conviction.

Her parents, listening attentively to her thoughtful words, became increasingly sure of their daughter's commitment to the relationship. At this moment, they felt a surge of pride, realizing they had raised a child who believed in the essence of relationships, unburdened by societal expectations. They willingly approved of Simran's choice, assuring her of their support, and eagerly extended an invitation to Vinay for a dinner where the bonds of the two families would intertwine.

The approaching weekend brought Vinay to Simran's house, where he was greeted with warmth and the expressed desire of Simran's family to welcome him as their son-in-law. The surprise overwhelmed Vinay, catching him off guard, as Simran had orchestrated this special moment without giving him a heads-up. In the midst of the familial joy, tears of happiness welled up in Vinay's eyes, making it a day he had never experienced before.

Amidst the conversations and shared laughter, Vinay, grateful for the moment but with a sense of responsibility, expressed his plans. He explained that since his recent promotion and the decision to buy a house, he had certain responsibilities toward his family. While he cherished the prospect of becoming a part of Simran's family, he requested some time to fulfill his familial obligations before taking the next step in their relationship.

The next day, Simran's parents, brimming with happiness, paid a visit to Vinay's family. The atmosphere was charged with the anticipation of discussing the chance for an upcoming engagement ceremony. Seated together, they exchanged pleasantries before diving into the details. Simran's parents, knowing Vinay's family well and having witnessed Vinay's dedication, felt confident in this alliance. Vinay's family, equally pleased with the match, enthusiastically embraced the idea of an engagement, appreciating the significance of celebrating this milestone in the couple's journey.

As the conversation progressed, the families decided on a date, fixing the engagement ceremony exactly after 88 days. Both Simran and Vinay, overjoyed by the unanimous agreement, couldn't wait for the special day to arrive. Their families, now connected by this upcoming celebration, shared laughter and stories, further strengthening the bond between them.

Simran, unable to contain her excitement, snapped a photo with Vinay, capturing the essence of their joy. Without delay, she posted the picture on social media, crafting a heartfelt caption that announced their engagement. In a playful touch, she tagged Vijay and Vaibhav, the friends who had been part of their journey from the beginning, adding the word "surprise" to evoke curiosity and share the news in a way that mirrored the camaraderie they all cherished. The post quickly garnered comments and likes, echoing the shared happiness of their extended social circle.

Vijay, just stepping into his home, glanced at his phone and caught sight of Simran's engagement announcement. His face lit up with joy, and without a second thought, he rushed over to Vinay's place.

Vijay's excitement bubbled over as he entered Vinay's home. "Vinay, my man! Congratulations!" he exclaimed, still holding his friend in a hearty embrace. Vinay, caught off guard by the sudden intrusion, couldn't help but laugh at Vijay's infectious enthusiasm. "Thanks, Vijay! I'm glad you came over," Vinay replied, reciprocating the hug. They both knew that Vijay was as much a part of this journey as anyone.

In the midst of the celebration, Vinay decided to give Vaibhav a call, knowing how absorbed he could get in his work. Vaibhav, focused on his tasks, answered the call with a casual "Hey, what's up?" Unveiling the surprise, Vijay guided Vaibhav to check Simran's latest social media post. As Vaibhav saw the announcement, his initial reaction was a dramatic "Whaaaaaat!" The surprise in his voice resonated through the phone, and laughter erupted on the other end. "You're unbelievable, Vaibhav!" Vijay teased.

Despite the distance, the trio shared a moment of camaraderie, with Vaibhav promising to join the celebration the next day. The anticipation of the impending get-together filled the air, and the excitement was palpable even through the phone.

The next day, Vinay, Vijay, and Vaibhav gathered at a cozy restaurant, eagerly waiting for Simran to join them. The air buzzed with excitement, and the atmosphere was filled with the anticipation of celebration.

As Vinay and Simran walked hand in hand, their joy radiated, setting a lively tone for the gathering. Vaibhav, observing his friends' happiness, felt a warm emotional tug, realizing the value of companionship and shared joys in life. The trio greeted Simran with cheerful smiles and exchanged affectionate hugs.

The conversation flowed seamlessly, with laughter and anecdotes from their individual journeys over the past few years. Vinay shared the subsequent success in his career, while Vijay talked about his diverse experiences in content curation. Vaibhav, despite the challenges of his entrepreneurial journey, found solace in the genuine happiness of his friends.

Amidst the storytelling and laughter, Vaibhav couldn't help but express his emotions. "You know, guys, seeing both of you so happy together makes me realize the importance of having a companion. Someone with whom I can share all the happenings in my life," he confessed, a hint of vulnerability in his voice.

Understanding Vaibhav's sentiments, Vinay and Vijay assured him of their unwavering support. "We're always here for you, Vaibhav. Friends are like family, and we're in this together," Vinay affirmed, echoing the sentiment shared by all three.

Simran, sensing the emotional moment, chimed in, "Absolutely! Friendship is not just about sharing joys but also being there for each other in tougher times. We're a team, and we'll always be."

With that heartfelt exchange, they raised their glasses for a toast, a symbol of the enduring bond they shared. The clinking of glasses echoed in the restaurant as they cheered not just for the present moment but for the beginnings of many more celebrations in the journey of their intertwined lives.

Takeaways:

★ Advocate for the normalization and prioritization of mental health in society.

★ Emphasize equality and shared responsibilities as foundations for successful marriages.

★ Address challenges related to familial expectations and personal choices.

★ Promote the idea that companionship and mutual support are essential aspects of a successful relationship.

★ Encourage professionals to expand their roles to provide holistic guidance.

★ Foster an environment of unwavering support and celebration of each other's successes.

Chapter 11
Milestones and Unveiled Journeys

"One must believe in making a difference, no matter how small. If each one of us contributes positively, the impact can be significant."

On the agreed-upon date, the much-anticipated moment arrived for Vinay and Simran—their engagement day. Meanwhile, Vaibhav, who had been diligently immersing himself in the fashion industry, had seamlessly incorporated his expertise into his family's business with the support of his friends. Over the past month, he has introduced innovative methods and embraced current market trends and demands.

Recognizing Vaibhav's exceptional capabilities, Simran and Vinay decided to choose outfits from his firm, and the results were nothing short of fabulous. The couple enjoyed a beautiful day filled with love and celebration, and their engagement photoshoot caught the attention of multiple press release channels. Vaibhav's efforts in delivering the perfect attire for his friends garnered recognition, proving that Vinay's words about life preparing Vaibhav for something big were coming true.

Vijay extended his heartfelt congratulations to the happy couple and, recognizing Vaibhav's dedication and success, expressed his appreciation. The day concluded with laughter echoing in the air, dreams taking flight for the newly engaged couple, and hopes soaring for Vaibhav's future endeavors. As they embraced the promising journey ahead, the trio found comfort in the strength of their friendship, each contributing in their own way to the their shared moments and collective achievements.

In the quiet moments after a long day, Vijay found himself in his bedroom, genuinely happy for Simran and Vinay. The door creaked open, and Mr. Singh, Vijay's father, entered the room to check on his son.

"Vijay, are you okay?" Mr. Singh inquired. Surprised by the unexpected question, Vijay replied, "Yes, Dad, I'm fine, but I didn't get the intention." Mr. Singh then revealed that he was aware of Vijay's feelings toward Simran. While happy for Vinay and Simran, as a concerned father, he wanted to ensure Vijay was doing well.

"Thanks, Dad, but I'm absolutely fine," Vijay assured him. "Yes, I did like Simran, and I still do, but I don't want to label the emotion. I am her friend and her well-wisher, and she is the same for me. We will always be the same, but this doesn't necessarily demand a romantic relationship. I'm genuinely happy for my friends, and I am totally okay with it."

Mr. Singh then probed, "Are you planning to see a girl?" Vijay responded, "No, Dad, at this point, I would like to go with the family's choice. However, I'm open to meeting the girl to get to know her before committing to marriage." Mr. Singh, pleased with his son's mature response, suggested a girl from his wife's relatives whom they believed to be a suitable match. Vijay agreed to meet her.

Seeing Vijay embrace life, unfazed by the developments around him, proved that he was indeed mature. His perspective on love, recognizing it in various forms without the need for ownership, showcased his understanding of relationships.

The following month, Vijay had the opportunity to meet Anita, the girl suggested by his family. They engaged in heartfelt conversations, discovering shared interests and values that formed the foundation of a potential connection. As they spent more time together, Vijay found Anita's genuine nature and kind spirit to be truly endearing. Anita, in turn, appreciated Vijay's calm demeanor and thoughtful approach to life. In the midst of these shared moments, they realized that their connection was deepening.

As the topic of marriage gradually surfaced, Anita expressed her genuine interest in building a life with Vijay. In a candid conversation, she shared her thoughts on love, family, and the importance of mutual respect in a relationship. Vijay, recognizing the sincerity in Anita's words and feeling a sense of resonance with her values, decided to take this significant step in his life.

The announcement of their decision brought immense joy to both families. Vijay's parents, having witnessed their son's mature and thoughtful approach, welcomed Anita with open arms. The once-tense atmosphere that had lingered due to differences of opinion within the family now seemed to dissipate, replaced by a shared happiness and excitement for Vijay's impending marriage.

The discussions surrounding the wedding became a bridge that connected family members, allowing them to appreciate the beauty of new beginnings and the bonds that tie them together. The once-strained relationships found healing in the warmth of this shared joy, marking a turning point for the family, who now looked forward to celebrating not just Vijay and Anita's union but the unity and understanding that had grown within their own hearts.

As the relationship between Vijay and Anita solidified, Vijay eagerly introduced Anita to his circle of friends, including Vinay and Simran. The bond between the friends expanded, and Simran found in Anita not just a future sister-in-law but a new friend in town. Anita's warm and kind-hearted nature quickly endeared her to everyone.

With every passing day, Anita became an integral part of the close-knit group. Her friendly demeanor and genuine interest in the lives of each friend endeared her even more to Simran, Vinay, and the others.

One day, as they all gathered for dinner, Vijay couldn't help but express his joy at how seamlessly Anita had become a part of their lives. "I'm so glad you all get along well. It means a lot to me," Vijay said, looking at Anita with a grateful smile. Anita, in turn, replied, "Your friends are amazing. I feel blessed to be a part of such a wonderful group."

Simran, always perceptive, chimed in, "Anita, we're not just friends; we're family. And family always grows; it welcomes new members with open arms." Vinay nodded in agreement, adding, "Absolutely, Anita. We've seen each other through thick and thin, and having you here feels just right."

The conversation shifted to the future, with everyone sharing their aspirations and dreams. Anita, with her intelligence, bravery, and empathy, proved to be a perfect match for Vijay. Her involvement with NGOs dedicated to upholding small-scale industries showcased her commitment to social causes. Anita, with her dedication to social causes, spoke passionately about her work with NGOs. "I believe in making a difference, no matter how small. If each one of us contributes positively, the impact can be significant," she shared.

The lives of these friends were now evolving into a new dimension, marked by individual progress and the anticipation of joyous new beginnings for each of them. Within a year, Vinay's journey had come full circle when he finally took possession of the keys to his own apartment.

The significance of this moment wasn't lost on him or those close to him. For a family that had experienced the challenges of compromise while living in a rented house, owning their own space was a dream realized.

The day was filled with mixed emotions—a blend of pride, joy, and a sense of accomplishment. Vinay stood in the doorway of his new home, reflecting on the years of hard work, determination, and sacrifices that had led to this moment. His family, too, shared in his happiness, feeling the warmth of a place they could truly call their own.

Simran, Vijay, and Vaibhav, who had been witnesses to Vinay's journey, celebrated this milestone with him. As they stepped into the freshly acquired abode, Simran remarked, "Vinay, you've turned this place into a haven. It's not just a house; it's a testament to your dedication and perseverance." Vijay added, "This is more than bricks and mortar; it's a symbol of your success and the love you have for your family."

Vaibhav, recognizing the significance of the moment, noted, "Vinay, you've not just built a house; you've built a home filled with memories waiting to be made. This is an achievement for all of us."

The group shared laughter and stories, appreciating the journey that had brought them to this point. Vinay's new home wasn't just a structure; it was a tangible representation of dreams fulfilled and the unwavering support of friends and family. The warmth of shared celebrations lingered in the air, marking the beginning of a new chapter for Vinay and his loved ones.

As the symbolic key to Vinay's new apartment opened the door to a new chapter in his life, the wedding plans fell into place with meticulous timing. The couple, Vinay and Simran, envisioned not just a wedding but the commencement of their shared life within the walls of their new home. Despite everyone's hectic schedules, the friends rallied together to ensure that the wedding preparations were a collective effort.

Anita, Vijay's soon-to-be wife, also joined in to contribute her part, turning the wedding preparations into a shared venture among the close-knit group. The camaraderie that had defined their friendship now translated seamlessly into the collaborative effort to create a memorable wedding.

The ceremony was a blend of traditions and modern aspirations, a reflection of Vinay and Simran's journey. The exchange of vows echoed not only the commitment between the couple but also the shared dreams they aspired to fulfill in their new life together. The support of friends and family was palpable, turning the celebration into a joyous occasion filled with laughter, love, and shared hopes for the future.

As Vinay and Simran embarked on this new chapter, the walls of their new home witnessed the beginning of a life intertwined with shared dreams, responsibilities, and the warmth of love. The close proximity of the wedding to Vinay's home ownership added an extra layer of significance to the celebrations, marking the start of a journey that promised to be as unique and special as the couple themselves.

Takeaways:

★ Encourage entrepreneurs to incorporate innovative methods and stay updated on market trends.

★ Highlight the importance of shared efforts in creating memorable life events.

★ Promote the idea that friends and family play a crucial role in supporting and enriching relationships.

★ Encourage shared aspirations and dreams within support circles to strengthen bonds.

★ Highlight the significance of a home as more than a physical structure.

Chapter 12

Harmony in Choices

"Life should be more than just chasing after material success."

In the midst of happy events, Vijay's wedding was just around the corner, adding to the joy felt by everyone. The happiness grew even more when it was revealed that Vijay had earned a promotion to become the head of a branch, showing how much he had progressed in his job. This brought excitement not only to Vijay and Anita but also to their families.

During the celebrations, Mr. Singh, Vijay's father, was thinking about something important. Reflecting on his own life and seeing Vijay's success, he felt comfortable considering an early retirement. The idea of enjoying life at a slower pace seemed appealing, and he was confident in handing over responsibilities to the younger generation.

As Vijay and Anita got married, Mr. Singh and his wife decided to go back to their hometown. This wasn't just a break but a choice to enjoy the simple joys of life and reconnect with their roots. They left behind an open space, not in their absence, but to create room for the newlyweds to build their lives together.

In the midst of growing his business, Vaibhav found himself dealing with a mix of feelings. Even though his family was actively looking for potential matches among their business contacts, Vaibhav had his own unique preferences. While he greatly respected women who pursued careers, deep down, he desired a different kind of companionship—someone who would make a home. Maybe he wanted the soothing comfort of constant care—a place to find solace after a tiring day. For Vaibhav, choosing a partner who preferred homemaking was a personal decision, something he felt didn't need explaining. He believed it was about different ways of looking at things, and he thought that every choice deserved understanding and acceptance.

A few months passed, and life continued its smooth course for everyone. Recognizing Vaibhav's potential and after careful consideration, his father officially announced him as the next head of their family business. It was a title well-earned by Vaibhav, marking a significant milestone in his professional journey. To celebrate this achievement, a small party was organized, attended by Vinay and Vijay along with their wives.

The party became a gathering where relatives and well-wishers offered bridal suggestions for Vaibhav, given that he was now settled in his personal life. Among the attendees were also Vaibhav's colleagues from his startup. Their company had successfully made a mark in the market, largely due to Vaibhav's significant contributions. His adept business skills not only propelled the company forward but also reflected in how he retained people and fostered strong relationships. The celebration marked not just a career milestone for Vaibhav but also a testament to the impact he had on those around him.

In the quietude of that night, Vaibhav found himself immersed in profound contemplation about choosing his life partner. The question loomed large: should he opt for the one society deemed the best, or should he focus on the person who was best for him? As he scrolled through his news feed, a quote caught his eye, extolling the beauty of simple relationships. This resonated with Vaibhav, who was clear that he desired a connection where emotional investment took precedence over material considerations.

In the midst of this dilemma, he made a conscious decision. That night, he created a profile on a matrimonial site, simply as Vaibhav, setting out on a journey to explore and discover a relationship that aligned with his values and aspirations.

The following morning, Vaibhav found himself with a handful of prospects, yet none sparked his interest due to mismatched preferences. However, after a few days of scrolling through profiles, he stumbled upon one that caught his attention: Vidya. Although she was two years older than him, the compatibility in their preferences intrigued him. Taking the first step, he sent her a request, and as they engaged in a lengthy conversation, Vaibhav felt a growing inclination to explore the possibility of moving forward.

Vidya, with a background in working for an MNC, had accumulated significant financial independence over the years. However, she had reached a point where she questioned the conventional idea of the rat race and the practice of saving everything for retirement. Vidya, a wise investor, expressed her belief that life should be more than just chasing after material success. Financially secure, she revealed her interest in transitioning to a role as a homemaker, emphasizing her priorities centered around creating and nurturing a family. Her clarity of thought and independence without helplessness captivated Vaibhav the most.

Their decision to meet in person was met with anticipation and excitement. When Vaibhav and Vidya finally came face-to-face, Vaibhav was captivated by Vidya's positive approach and mindfulness. It was evident to him that she was someone who lived in the present, appreciating and savoring each moment of her life.

As the conversation deepened, Vaibhav revealed his identity and background, causing Vidya to be pleasantly surprised. Instead of being taken aback, she found his perspectives intriguing, and the revelation added a layer of complexity and depth to their budding connection. The more they shared their thoughts and beliefs, the clearer it became that they were in sync, and both of them felt a growing sense of compatibility.

As Vaibhav hailed from a joint family, he approached the matter conscientiously. Taking a step forward, he revealed to his family that he had connected with someone on a matrimonial site. The news brought happiness to his family, as they were glad to see Vaibhav finally on board with the idea of marriage. However, a subtle concern arose among them: Vidya was older than Vaibhav.

This concern lingered as the family agreed to meet Vidya, albeit with some reservations. Despite the initial hesitation, Vaibhav's confidence and Vidya's warm aura managed to win over the hearts of his joint family. Eventually, they gave their approval, albeit with a condition—that Vidya's age would not be disclosed to society during the wedding. This compromise allowed Vaibhav to move forward with the support of his family, setting the stage for a unique and meaningful union.

Initially, Vaibhav was conscious of Vidya's reaction, but to his relief, she demonstrated a deep understanding that compromising on certain aspects, which were not inherently harmful, was sometimes necessary. Vidya recognized that societies operated within established norms, and challenging them at every step might not always yield positive results. She advocated for patience and the gradual evolution of perspectives.

Vidya, being wise beyond her years, accepted the condition without hesitation, acknowledging the delicate balance between personal choices and societal expectations. This understanding between them laid the foundation for a harmonious partnership. As a result, Vaibhav and Vidya were happily married within the span of the next three months, embarking on a journey that embraced their individuality while navigating the complexities of societal norms.

Takeaways:

★ Highlight the importance of balancing personal and professional lives.

★ Advocate for reconnecting with roots and exploring simpler joys in life.

★ Encourage individuals to reflect on their personal values when choosing life partners.

★ Advocate for financial independence, allowing individuals to make choices beyond the conventional rat race.

★ Encourage couples to embrace their individuality in marriages.

Shades of Life

Chapter 13
A Journey Into Life Coaching

"Sometimes, the biggest leaps are taken not alone but hand in hand with those who believe in the journey."

As the next two years passed, a sense of peace and contentment enveloped everyone's lives. Vinay and Simran were on the brink of a new chapter, expecting their first child. Meanwhile, Vinay and Vijay found themselves engaged in a collaborative project between their companies. The project focused on launching an AI software product designed to assist people in their daily lives.

During this collaboration, Vijay keenly observed Vinay's exceptional skills in understanding people and providing thoughtful solutions. Upon the successful launch of the AI product, Vijay had a revelation. He suggested to Vinay that he should consider life coaching, given his innate ability to connect with people and offer valuable guidance. Vinay, upon reflection, realized that he had been unknowingly practicing elements of life coaching in his interactions.

In a moment of camaraderie, Vijay even recounted the incident when Vinay had motivated Vaibhav, highlighting Vinay's natural inclination towards guiding and motivating others. Vinay appreciated Vijay's insightful suggestion and felt grateful for the encouragement to explore a new dimension in his career.

Vinay, despite the appeal of Vijay's suggestion about life coaching, found himself grappling with skepticism. The prospect of a career change posed a significant challenge, considering the responsibilities resting on his shoulders. Simran was pregnant, Vinay's sister had chosen to pursue higher studies, and his parents were dependent on him for support. In this complex web of familial obligations, the idea of venturing into a new career seemed like a risky decision.

Vijay, perceptive to Vinay's predicament, chose not to press the matter further. However, recognizing Vinay's potential, Vijay decided to discuss the idea with Simran. He shared his insights into Vinay's exceptional skills and the potential success he could achieve as a life coach. Simran, understanding the importance of supporting Vinay's aspirations, agreed with Vijay's perspective.

Determined to help her husband explore new opportunities, Simran promised Vijay that she would talk to Vinay and express her support for his potential career change.

One evening, as they sat together at home, Simran gently broached the topic.

"Vinay, I had an interesting conversation with Vijay today," she said.

"Oh? About what?"

"About you, actually. He sees great potential in you as a life coach."

Vinay, smiling at Simran, said, "Yes, he told the same to me too, Simran."

"Yes, and you know what? I agree with him. You have this amazing ability to understand people and guide them positively. I think it could be a fulfilling career for you."

Vinay looked skeptical.

"I appreciate that, Simran, but it's a big leap. I have responsibilities, especially now with you being pregnant, my sister's education, and our parents."

"I completely understand, Vinay. But what if we approach it gradually? You don't have to take a huge risk right away. How about considering a course in life coaching and practicing it alongside your current job? It might be a good way to test the waters."

"That actually sounds reasonable. I can learn and start practicing, and if it gains traction, maybe I can think about a career shift later."

"Exactly! We can take it step by step, and I'm here to support you in every decision. What do you think?"

"Alright, let's give it a shot. I appreciate your support, Simran."

Vinay's journey as a life coach unfolded with remarkable success. Over the course of a year, he not only completed his coaching course but also began actively working with clients. Simran played a significant role in providing him with opportunities and introducing him to some of her clients. Additionally, Vijay and Vaibhav, recognizing Vinay's mentoring abilities, enlisted his expertise to train their colleagues.

The support from his friends and family was instrumental in Vinay's growing confidence. He extended his mentorship beyond the corporate world, collaborating with Anita's NGO to contribute to the growth of small-scale businesses. Vinay's reputation as a skilled life coach and mentor continued to flourish, leading to invitations from various sectors.

As Vinay dedicated himself to coaching individuals and guiding small industries, he made the decision to resign from his corporate job. However, recognizing his valuable contribution, his company offered him the role of training their employees—a testament to his exemplary skills as a mentor.

Throughout this challenging period, Simran's unwavering support was a pillar of strength for Vinay. Despite the crucial time, she ensured minimal disruptions, even giving birth to twins during this period. Vinay found stability not only in his career but also in his newfound sense of contentment with his growing family. Grateful for the support of Simran and his friends, Vinay reflected on the transformative journey that led him to a fulfilling and balanced life.

Takeaways:

★ Highlight the potential for personal and professional growth through collaborative initiatives.

★ Encourage mentorship and support for those considering career changes.

★ Encourage open communication between spouses about career goals and aspirations.

★ Advocate for individuals to consider courses and skill development programs when contemplating career changes.

★ Encourage companies to recognize and value the skills of employees, even in different roles.

Chapter 14

Rooted in Love

"A life partner who not only complements your ambitions but also enriches your life with positivity and unwavering support is a treasure."

Vijay's journey of excellence reached a pinnacle when he was offered the role of CEO for a company, marking a significant milestone in his career. He had waited long enough to reach this position and the wait was worth it. The announcement ceremony was attended by his family, including Mr. and Mrs. Singh and Anita. It was a moment of immense pride, especially for Mr. Singh, who couldn't hold back tears of joy at seeing his son achieve such remarkable success. For a father, seeing his child follow in his footsteps and excel in their career is a source of immeasurable pride.

Vijay, being the reflection of his father's early career success, understood the depth of this moment for Mr. Singh. It was a beautiful reminder of the legacy and values passed down through generations. As Vijay assumed the role of CEO, he brought his leadership skills to the forefront, taking the company to new heights and solidifying his reputation as a dynamic and visionary leader.

Vijay's collaboration with Vinay proved to be a game-changer as they introduced innovative techniques in their company. Together, they built a cohesive team that not only excelled in internal collaborations but also attracted international clients who outsourced their content needs. The synergy between Vijay and Vinay was evident as they navigated the challenges and opportunities in the industry.

Vijay's visionary approach led to the introduction of his own software, revolutionizing content generation. This groundbreaking discovery created waves in the industry, establishing Vijay as an unstoppable force. His influence extended beyond the boundaries of his company, making him one of the most influential figures in the corporate world. Vijay's expertise was sought after, and he found himself frequently invited as a chief guest at various industry events, further solidifying his reputation as a leader and innovator.

In that special function at the children's school, Vijay took the stage as the guest of honor, warmly sharing his experiences and insights with the audience. The crowd was captivated by his words, and Anita stood by, proud of the person Vijay had become. The couple's commitment to each other was evident, not just in the public eye but in the quiet moments at the end of each day when they made time for each other.

After the event, in the serenity of their home, Vijay expressed a deep desire to become a father. Anita, thoughtful and introspective, responded with her perspective on the notion of expanding their family. She carefully articulated that while the idea of having a biological child had crossed her mind, she was strongly considering the option of adoption. For Anita, every child, regardless of their biological connection, deserved love, care, and a nurturing environment. In her eyes, adoption represented a meaningful way to contribute to society and provide a loving home to a child in need.

Vijay, taking in Anita's heartfelt words, found resonance with her perspective. The idea of adoption struck a chord with him, aligning with their shared values of compassion and societal responsibility. The couple who are inclined toward family planning in the initial days of the marriage, were in agreement to have one biological child and another child being the adopted one. This decision marked a beautiful chapter in their journey, rooted in love, empathy, and a shared commitment to building a family based on principles of care and inclusivity.

The next few months for Vijay and Anita were a rollercoaster of emotions, anticipation, and careful planning. Armed with the doctor's recommendations, the couple embarked on a journey of baby planning that would soon lead to the most transformative experience of their lives.

Vijay, always the meticulous planner, made sure they followed a balanced lifestyle. From nutrition to exercise, he was determined to provide the best possible environment for Anita and their soon-to-be baby. Anita, on the other hand, embraced the changes with grace and resilience, trusting Vijay's lead and relishing the excitement of impending motherhood.

As the days turned into weeks and the weeks into months, the couple's efforts bore fruit. Anita discovered that they were expecting their first child. The news brought a flood of emotions—joy, excitement, and a touch of nervousness. Parenthood was a new chapter, and they were eager to embrace it with open hearts.

The journey of pregnancy was a mixed bag of emotions for Anita. The glow on her face and the growing baby bump were constant reminders of the life growing within her. However, the experience also came with its own set of challenges, from morning sickness to mood swings. Vijay stood by her side, offering support and understanding through it all.

Preparing for the arrival of their little one became a joint venture. The couple attended prenatal classes, read parenting books, and set up a cozy nursery. Vijay meticulously assembled baby furniture, while Anita added personal touches to make the space warm and welcoming.

As the due date approached, the couple found themselves reflecting on the journey they had undertaken. They had faced challenges, learned together, and grown as a couple. The anticipation and nervousness were replaced by a deep sense of readiness and excitement.

When the day finally arrived, the labor room echoed with a mix of tension and joy. Vijay held Anita's hand, offering words of encouragement and support. The cries of their newborn filled the room, marking the beginning of a new chapter in their lives.

Parenthood brought with it sleepless nights, endless diaper changes, and a newfound level of responsibility. Yet, amidst the challenges, Vijay and Anita found profound joy in the simple moments—the first smile, the sound of tiny laughter, and the warmth of a tiny body nestled in their arms.

In the end, the couple managed to turn the challenges of parenthood into opportunities for growth and connection. The sleepless nights became shared moments of bonding, and the challenges strengthened their partnership.

The following five years unfolded in a blur of laughter, diaper changes, and countless bedtime stories for Anita and Vijay. Devoting themselves wholeheartedly to the upbringing of their child, they made sure she was surrounded by love, care, and a world filled with endless possibilities.

As their little one's fifth birthday approached, the house buzzed with excitement. The living room was adorned with colorful decorations, and a homemade birthday cake sat proudly on the table. Friends and family gathered to celebrate the milestone, sharing in the joy of watching their beloved child grow.

Amidst the laughter and festivities, a well-intentioned relative chimed in, "She needs a little playmate, don't you think? Time for another one?" The suggestion hung in the air, prompting Anita and Vijay to exchange knowing glances.

The idea of expanding their family had been a quiet promise between them since the early days of their marriage. However, it wasn't about biology or blood; it was about creating a home filled with love and companionship. Adoption had always been a part of their shared vision, a promise they made to each other when they embarked on this journey of parenthood.

As they smiled at each other, it was a silent acknowledgment of that promise. The relative's words had brought to the surface a plan that had been quietly taking shape in their hearts. The couple had always believed in the power of love to create a family, and the time felt right to fulfill their commitment to adoption.

In the weeks that followed, Anita and Vijay began exploring the possibilities of adoption. They navigated paperwork, attended adoption seminars, and opened their hearts to the idea of welcoming another child into their lives. The process was not without its challenges, but the couple faced them with the same determination and love that had defined their parenting journey so far.

Months later, the day arrived when they met their new family member—a child who had been waiting for a loving home. The laughter in their household multiplied, bedtime stories became a shared adventure, and the little one seamlessly became a part of the love-filled world Anita and Vijay had created.

As they celebrated their daughter's sixth birthday, surrounded by the warmth of family and the laughter of two siblings, Anita and Vijay couldn't help but marvel at the journey they had undertaken. The past six years have been a testament to their commitment to each other and their shared dream of building a family bound not by blood but by the unbreakable bonds of love and devotion.

Vijay and Anita embraced their roles as parents wholeheartedly, ensuring that all parental duties were met with love and dedication. Mr. and Mrs. Singh, proud grandparents, made it a point to visit the family twice a year. While they typically spent the majority of the year in their native place, the presence of the children at home became a delightful reason for extending their stay with Vijay and Anita.

The child quickly adapted to its new surroundings, forming strong bonds with the adoptive parents and grandparents. The household echoed with the laughter and playful banter of the youngsters, creating an atmosphere of warmth and familial love. Vijay found that his life was now lived with a distinct purpose, not only in his professional endeavors but also in the enriching experiences of parenthood.

Takeaways:

★ Establish a forum for professionals to collaborate on innovative projects, fostering creativity and cross-industry partnerships.

★ Develop a toolkit on work-life balance, providing practical tips, resources, and strategies for maintaining a healthy balance in personal and professional life.

★ Advocate for adoption awareness by organizing events, sharing success stories, and dispelling myths surrounding adoption to promote inclusivity.

★ Create wellness challenges that focus on balanced lifestyles, incorporating elements of nutrition, exercise, and mental well-being for holistic health.

★ Encourage community service initiatives by supporting local organizations, NGOs, and charitable causes, fostering a sense of social responsibility and contribution.

★ Conduct workshops on financial literacy, empowering individuals to make informed decisions about budgeting, investing, and achieving financial goals.

★ Establish an entrepreneurship incubator to support aspiring entrepreneurs, providing resources, mentorship, and networking opportunities.

Chapter 15

Beyond Biology

"Parenthood is not confined to biology; it's a journey of love, care, and societal responsibility—rooted in compassion."

In the vibrant city of Mumbai, amidst the hustle and bustle of urban life, Vaibhav's multiple outlets served as hubs for his entrepreneurial endeavors. However, amid the demanding challenges of managing business ventures, Vaibhav discovered a sanctuary in the form of Vidya, his life partner. Vidya, with her innate ability to seamlessly take charge of household responsibilities, not only became an integral part of Vaibhav's life but also won the affection of every family member.

Vidya's positive aura and good-natured demeanor became the hallmarks of her presence within the family. Her dedication as a wife was unwavering, and her compatibility with Vaibhav was evident in their harmonious relationship. What set Vidya apart was her unique skill of balancing family responsibilities while retaining her individual identity. This resonated deeply with Vaibhav, who found a sense of completeness in her companionship.

Vidya's presence filled the subtle gaps in Vaibhav's life, bringing a newfound richness to their shared moments. As they navigated the intricacies of daily life together, their journey as life partners became woven with fulfillment and joy. Whether spending quality time amidst the comforting walls of their home or facing the challenges of the bustling city, Vaibhav and Vidya embraced each experience, creating a life of shared purpose and contentment.

Living in a joint family brought its own set of unique dynamics and challenges, yet Vaibhav and Vidya willingly embraced this environment, recognizing the inherent beauty in shared experiences and connections. As days turned into weeks and weeks into years, the couple found themselves amidst societal expectations, particularly those related to starting a family.

Despite the constant inquiries from well-meaning relatives and acquaintances, the couple faced a stark reality. Even after two years of marriage, Vidya could not conceive. This revelation hit them hard, casting a shadow of disappointment and sadness. In navigating this unexpected turn of events, Vaibhav, aware of the various perspectives within their joint family, became a pillar of support for Vidya.

Understanding the nuances of societal expectations and familial dynamics, Vaibhav ensured that Vidya did not bear the weight of this revelation alone. In their quest for parenthood, Vaibhav and Vidya sought the guidance of medical professionals. After exploring various options, they decided on gestational surrogacy as the path to expanding their family. Vidya, understanding the emotional depth of motherhood, embraced the idea wholeheartedly, believing that the essence of being a mother transcended biological ties.

Choosing to keep this journey a closely guarded secret, the couple decided to create some distance from their extended family for a year. Vaibhav, a mastermind in orchestrating this delicate plan, revealed that Vidya was experiencing a challenging pregnancy and required specialized care. To ensure the success of their plan, the couple relocated to a different city, where they meticulously managed every aspect of the gestational surrogacy process.

During this period, Vaibhav continued his work remotely, skillfully concealing any hints of their true situation from their family. After a year of dedicated efforts, the couple returned triumphant, presenting their family with the gift of a healthy and happy baby. The arrival of their little one was met with joy and acceptance from the entire family, marking a poignant chapter in Vaibhav and Vidya's journey of resilience, love, and parenthood.

As the joyous atmosphere enveloped the family, Vidya couldn't help but ponder the path they had chosen. In that moment of subtle uncertainty, Vaibhav, attuned to his wife's unspoken thoughts, reassured her with a comforting gesture. He affirmed that the decisions they had made were indeed right for their family.

Vidya, despite not giving physical birth to the child they had embraced, never felt a sense of inadequacy. The couple shared a profound understanding that transcended biological ties. They believed in the power of emotion and love, dismissing the notion that motherhood is solely defined by genetics. In their eyes, Vidya was already a mother, nurturing a connection that went beyond biological intricacies.

Choosing to keep the details of the gestational surrogacy private, Vaibhav and Vidya witnessed the happiness of their family flourishing. They held a conviction that, as long as their actions brought joy without causing harm, maintaining a level of secrecy was justified. Over time, the couple found themselves living the life they had envisioned—surrounded by their complete family, bound by love, understanding, and the shared joy of their unconventional yet deeply fulfilling journey.

Takeaways:

★ Create support groups for entrepreneurs to share experiences and strategies for balancing work and personal life.

★ Launch campaigns to raise awareness about alternative paths to parenthood like natural surrogacy, IVF, promoting inclusivity and breaking societal stereotypes.

★ Conduct seminars and discussions on redefining parenthood, emphasizing the importance of emotional connections over biological ties.

★ Develop workshops on maintaining family harmony while embracing unconventional life choices, promoting open dialogue and understanding.

★ Advocate for inclusive parenthood initiatives, encouraging society to recognize and celebrate diverse paths to building loving families.

Concluding Note

As we conclude our journey with Vinay, Vijay, and Vaibhav in this 21st century, it's evident that life, much like a winding river, can take various courses. Each of our characters embarked on their own unique paths, traversing the landscape of life with distinct approaches that reflected their individual philosophies.

Vinay, driven by his idealistic vision, viewed life through the lens of grand aspirations and noble ideals. His approach was marked by a commitment to lofty principles, navigating the intricate dance of existence with a heart full of dreams. Vinay's journey unfolded as a series of steps toward an envisioned future, always mindful of the greater purpose and the impact of each calculated move on the canvas of his ideals.

Vijay, the astute and adaptive thinker, embraced life as a playground of intellect and adaptability. His sharp mind allowed him to navigate the complexities of life with a blend of intelligence and resourcefulness. Rather than adhering to a predefined plan, Vijay thrived on taking calculated risks and seizing opportunities that presented themselves. His journey unfolded like a well-played chess game, with strategic moves and the wisdom to adapt to the ever-changing dynamics.

Vaibhav, a person of undeniable strengths and occasional flaws, approached life with a steady and patient demeanor. His journey was a testament to the ebb and flow of resilience and determination. While facing life's challenges, Vaibhav's quiet strength came to the forefront, relying on perseverance to overcome obstacles. Acknowledging his imperfections, Vaibhav's journey became a relatable tale of navigating the highs and lows with a genuine, flawed, and authentic spirit.

Life is this intricate masterpiece, and within its threads, you find Vinay, Vijay, and Vaibhav each contributing a distinct hue. They're not just characters; they're the brushstrokes that add depth and richness to the collective canvas of our shared narrative. Their diverse approaches are like different shades, reflecting the vast spectrum of the human experience.

Together, they form this kaleidoscope of experiences, showcasing that success isn't a one-size-fits-all affair. It's a mosaic painted with varied strokes, a reminder that achievement can wear different faces and be seen through various lenses. The richness of life lies in embracing these diverse approaches and appreciating the beauty they bring to our collective story.

Beyond the trio, the story also unfolded through the lens of their wives and families, each contributing a unique perspective to the narrative. The diverse approaches of these families showcased the myriad ways people navigate the complexities of life, finding success and contentment through their own methods.

Life, as depicted in this tale, is not a one-size-fits-all experience. The characters, with their varied approaches, demonstrate that success and fulfillment are subjective concepts, shaped by individual perspectives and choices. The wives, families, and friends of Vinay, Vijay, and Vaibhav each played a role in adding depth and richness to the overarching story.

In the end, as we reflect on the lives of everyone, it becomes clear that diversity in approach does not hinder success. Despite their differences, each character successfully carved their own path, achieving personal and professional milestones in ways that resonated with their values and beliefs. Life, with its myriad approaches, is a tapestry woven with the threads of individual stories, each contributing to the beautiful mosaic of human experience.

Shades of Life

Epilogue

Thank you for embarking on this transformative journey with me through the pages of 'Shades of Life.' As the storyteller weaving the threads of these narratives, I discovered echoes of my own existence in the characters, and I hope you, too, found reflections of yourself in the diverse personalities presented. Each character, a unique shade in the canvas of life, offers the possibility of resonance with your own experiences.

In this book, I deliberately chose to illuminate positive and uplifting stories, steering clear of narratives that could potentially harm others in the pursuit of success. I believe in the power of positivity, and my intention was to inspire, uplift, and foster a sense of connection among our readers.

As a reader, have you encountered a character whose journey mirrors your own or evokes memories of decisions you wish you'd made differently in your early years? 'Shades of Life' is more than a mere collection of stories; it's an exploration of diverse approaches to life. Now, I'm intrigued: which personality resonated with you? Do you perceive the presented approaches as potential guides to enhance your own journey?

The decisions we make in life are deeply subjective. What works for one person may not work for the next. 'Shades of Life' does not provide a one-size-fits-all solution but rather challenges you to consider the various perspectives we encounter. The stories presented here are not instructions on how to live; instead, they reflect the myriad pathways individuals take on their unique journeys.

As you connect with the characters, recognize that the subjective approaches depicted are like the ebb and flow of life—dynamic, responsive to change, and not fixed in a rigid framework. These shifts signify growth, not compromise, as perspectives evolve with time and experience.

In crafting this narrative, my intention was not to prescribe a singular, correct approach. Instead, I aimed to create a mosaic of characters, each with their own set of joys, challenges, and triumphs, navigating life in their own authentic ways. Their stories echo the reality that life is complex, influenced by societal norms, personal choices, and the ever-shifting landscape.

The boundaries we set are often a product of our surroundings, and understanding this allows for adaptability and flexibility. In the grand symphony of existence, the diversity of approaches adds richness to the collective masterpiece. Happiness, measured by personal fulfillment, emerges as the true metric of success.

Let us cultivate a society that celebrates this diversity, acknowledging that every life, with its unique shades and experiences, contributes to the richness of the human experience. In doing so, we embrace the truth that each life is a work of art, beautiful in its own way. As we close this chapter, I encourage you to carry these narratives with you, contemplating the lessons they offer and perhaps finding inspiration in the hues of these life stories. After all, in the grand tapestry of existence, our individual stories weave together to create a rich and interconnected masterpiece.

About the Author

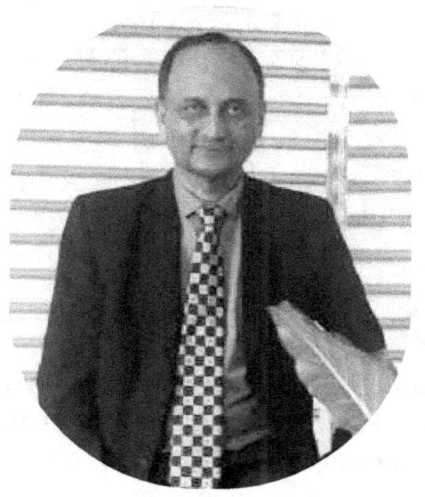

Dr. T. S. Parmar (PhD) is a distinguished professional with over 33 years of extensive experience in the Indian pharmaceutical industry. His academic prowess is marked by a Ph.D. in strategic management from Amity University and an honorary Ph.D. in marketing from Commonwealth Vocational University. Dr. Parmar has cultivated a robust academic background with a Master's in Marketing from Mumbai University, a Bachelor's in Life Sciences from St. Xavier's College (Mumbai University), and a BMCJ (Mass Communication & Journalism) from UTD Sagar.

A relentless pursuer of knowledge, Dr. Parmar has augmented his academic journey with prestigious courses such as the Executive Corporate Management Programme at IIM Ahmedabad and Senior Management Courses at ISB, Hyderabad. His commitment to advancing understanding in his field is exemplified by the release of his book, "Conceptual Understanding of the Indian Healthcare Industry" in 2021.

Demonstrating a holistic approach to learning, Dr. Parmar holds certifications in Reiki 1 and II and has completed courses in homeopathy (DOMH and DMMH) from a premier homeopathic institute in Chandigarh.

Throughout his illustrious career, Dr. Parmar has navigated diverse roles in leading MNCs and Indian pharmaceutical companies. His last position as the MD and CEO of Albert David Ltd. underscored his pivotal role in steering the company to success. His career trajectory spans various functional areas, including marketing, sales, strategy, M&As, and general management, positioning him as a key player in the industry.

Beyond his corporate achievements, Dr. Parmar actively contributes to academia. Serving as Visiting/Guest Faculty and as a member of the Board of Studies (BOS) and Board of Governors (BOG) at esteemed management institutes like Amity, Narsee Monjee, Lovely Professional University, and Ajeenkya D. Y. Patil University. He is passionate about imparting knowledge and experience. This commitment is further evident in his role as a keynote speaker, moderator, and panel member in conferences both in India and abroad.

Dr. Parmar's engagement extends beyond the professional realm. He is a proficient professional event anchor and host, also showcasing his communication skills as a voice-over artist. His eloquence is further demonstrated as a national-level debater. Outside the boardroom, Dr. Parmar is a versatile individual with a rich sporting background, excelling in junior national basketball, national yachting (enterprise class boat), and high-altitude trekking. He along with his wife has recently completed his challenging bucket list wish, Everest Base Camp [EBC] Trek in May'23. His diverse interests also include a fondness for music and dance, contributing to his well-rounded and dynamic personality.

Thank you for coming on the captivating journey through
"Shades of Life" by Dr. T. S. Parmar.
We're thrilled to have you as a reader!

Stay updated on all things related to the book
and Dr. T. S. Parmar
 Visit Our Website:
www.tsparmar.com

Scan the QR Code:

Exclusive Content and Updates

Book Launch News: Be the first to know about events, launches, and exclusive offers.

Behind the Scenes: Dive into the creative process with insights from Dr. T. S. Parmar.

Interactive Community: Join discussions, share your thoughts, and connect with fellow readers.

Thank you for being part of the Shades of Life community. Your support means the world to us!

Happy Reading!

www.ingramcontent.com/pod-product-compliance
Lightning Source LLC
LaVergne TN
LVHW010330070526
838199LV00065B/5707